A Comprehensive Guide to
Kundalini and Chakra Yog

A Comprehensive Guide to
Kundalini and Chakra Yog

Dr. Vishal Dwivedi

New Century Publications
New Delhi, India

NEW CENTURY PUBLICATIONS
74, Ansari Road, Ground Floor,
Daryaganj,
New Delhi - 110 002 (India)

Tel.: 011 - 4358 7398, 4101 7798, 2324 7798

Email: info@newcenturypublications.com

www.newcenturypublications.com

Editorial office:
4800/24, Bharat Ram Road,
Ansari Road, Daryaganj,
New Delhi – 110 002

Tel.: 98112 66355

Copyright © 2021 by the author

All rights reserved. No part of this book may be reproduced, stored in a retrieval system, or transmitted in any form or by any means, mechanical, photocopying, recording, or otherwise without the prior written permission of the publisher.

First Published: **2021**

ISBN: **978-81-7708-523-5**

Published by New Century Publications and printed at Milan Enterprises, New Delhi.

Designs: Patch Creative Unit, New Delhi.

PRINTED IN INDIA

Dedicated to

My Parents

About the Book

This book is about realizing the core of life—the energy which governs us to live, think, enact and react. The aim is to realize these energies and find the best alternatives for further growth. In Sanskrit, these confluence points are called *chakras* (wheels). In totality, a human body has 114 chakras—7 major chakras, 21 minor chakras and 86 micro chakras. 108 of them (including the 7 major ones) are more or less aimed towards the societal life and 6 of them towards the initial path of treading into the spiritual world.

Undoubtedly, a chakra is an energy centre. It is also a centre which coordinates the flow of energy within the body, thereby transmitting the energy to various organs and other confluence points—the other chakras. The unblocking of chakras is very crucial, rather it is paramount. The role of each chakra is important and its activation is equally significant.

Kundalini is a Sanskrit word, drawn from snakes, which when sleeps, tends to form a coil and drapes itself on it. It is a master energy of the body, through which the body can see things which are not visible and comprehend with things which are still unknown. For awakening of the kundalini, the nature and texture of the thoughts is vital.

The first step towards realising and opening up of the power house kundalini, is to balance the chakras in the body. Kundalini power is the ultimate power which can be attained by virtue of yog. Practicing yog postures, reciting mantras (in their correct texture, frequency and wavelengths), and breathing exercises are the most suitable ways to prepare body for the release of this energy. As is well-known, human body is made up of five elements, namely fire, ether, air, earth and water. Having an understanding of these five elements is primal before taking up yog or further advancing to the level of *kundalini yog*.

The present book focuses on 7 popular chakras, namely root chakra, solar plexus, sacral chakra, heart chakra, throat chakra, third eye chakra and the crown chakra.

About the Author

Dr. Vishal Dwivedi is a practicing Vedic psychologist with Ph.D. in Psychology and Masters in Yoga. Conscious of the fact that emotional and spiritual sides of an individual play a pivotal role in defining the personality traits, he has employed a unique blend of phonemes produced by *Vedic* Mantras and human emotions for healing purposes. The credit for his inclination towards spirituality goes to his mother Mrs. Santosh Dwivedi, who introduced him to spirituality at the tender age of five. She was instrumental in teaching him the primal essences of energy, derived from the five elements and imparting the skills of how these elements are generated, their behaviour and definition—what can be broadly classified as emotional, psychological, and physical aspects of life.

While embarking on the journey of *yog* and meditation, it is discernible to note that irrespective of the path or faith a person chooses, the tenets of life remain unaffected—designated as the elements. Interestingly, it is only the emotional part of the structure which can be altered and if an individual aspires to know and wishes to change the patterns of these elements, the approach has to be centered towards these elements only.

As part of the teachings advocated by his mother, the above approach should not be guided by man-made creations like language, religion, faith, systems and culture. Following this path as narrated by his mother and his extensive study and learning of the *Vedas* and their subsequent implementation in meditation, the author has been able to associate himself directly with the elements and the nature. Resultantly, he has developed a new technique to generate deficient hormone/chemicals, which are the primal causes of psychological or psychiatric ailments.

Contents

About the Book......vii
About the Author......viii
Preface......xi-xiii

1. **Kundalini Power: An Introduction** — 1-33

2. **Root Chakra: Mooldhara** — 34-52

3. **Manipura Chakra: Confluence of Fire, Water, Air and Earth Elements** — 53-74

4. **Swadisthana Chakra: Controlling the Water Element of the Body** — 75-96

5. **Anahata Chakra: The Confluence of Water, Earth, Fire, Air and Ether** — 97-117

6. **Vishudhi Chakra: Ether** — 118-137

7. **Agya Chakra: Space and Ether** — 138-158

8. **The Principles for Kundalini Awakening** — 159-172

Index — 173-177

Preface

An understanding about the core of life—the energy which governs us to live, think, enact and react—assumes significance to realize the dynamics and perceptions of life. The aim is to realize these energies and find the best alternatives for further growth. In Sanskrit, these confluence points are called *chakras* (wheels). In totality, there are 7 major chakras, 21 minor chakras and 86 micro chakras in a human body. Among the 114 chakras, 112 chakras reside within the body and the other 2, outside the body. Head, heart, navel, throat and base of the spine are the five main areas of major chakras. In contrast, the minor chakras are located in our hands, legs, tongue, knee, elbow, clavicles, shoulder, eye, ear and nose.

This book focuses on the seven popular chakras, namely root chakra, solar plexus, sacral chakra, heart chakra, throat chakra, third eye chakra and crown chakra. Chakra, undoubtedly, is an energy centre. It is also a centre which coordinates the flow of energy within the body, thereby transmitting the energy to various organs and other confluence points—the other chakras. It receives, assimilates and transmits the energy—the life force—to reach a point where you are able to go beyond the body and its other peripherals.

The unblocking of the chakras is very important, rather it is paramount. The role of each chakra is important and its activation is equally significant too. For the chakra to be able to heal itself there can be various paths which one may choose to tread. These could range from yog postures, to recitation of the mantras, to breathing exercises or to focus-based exercises. Basically, the chakras are portals between the inner and the outer world.

It has been long realised and found, that in human body, the power resides in the form of emotions and organ driving energies. However, in any of these states, the energy is unstable and keeps varying, while moving towards something else, either a place or a state, which this energy aspires to be in. Later, this state is realised, in which the energy is completely stable and progressive.

In Hindu scriptures, namely the *Vedas*, this is illustrated as the *shakti* aspiring to meet Shiva.

Kundalini is a Sanskrit word, drawn from snakes, which when sleeps, tends to form a coil and drapes itself on it. It is a master energy of the body, by which the body can see things which are not visible and know things which are still unknown. During the process of activation of kundalini, there is a huge release of energy, and due to this sudden release of energy, the human body is unable to hold onto to its conscious self most of the times. There are illustrations of what a *kundalini power* can do if and when activated, not only from the spiritual angle/facet but also in the sense of benefits that translate, for attaining greater gains in the societal world too.

For awakening of the kundalini, the nature and texture of your thoughts is vital. The first step towards realising and opening the power house kundalini, is to balance the chakras in the body. To experience pleasantness when kundalini is awakened, depends directly on the natural spectrum of energy with which one is born (the astrological natal chart). This is so because the blessings of the *shakti* can only be had with grace, as there is nothing which can allure her.

Kundalini movements are spontaneous, resembling certain *kriya(s)*—just like a wave pattern, which is not stable and rises and falls. Practicing yog postures, reciting mantras (in their correct texture, frequency and wavelengths), and breathing exercises are best ways to prepare the body for the release of this energy.

Post-realisation and activation of this serpentine power, the physical and behavioural personality of a person changes, inculcating and exhibiting a unique and differing kind of aura than the rest of the people around him/her.

In *Vedas*, the conduit for the energy to travel is called nadi which comes in varying shapes and sizes and amounts to 72,000 in number. It carries the energy from one chakra to another chakra and finally into the organs. By virtue of their significant role in the movement of energy, there are dedicated processes in yog, through which these nerves are kept clean and unblocked.

Kundalini power is the ultimate power which can be attained by virtue of yog as all other powers post-realisation of kundalini, cannot be achieved by performing yog. The powers travel across a person on their own as kundalini establishes a bridge between the cosmic and the ionic energy.

As is well-known, a human body is made up of five elements, namely fire, ether, air, earth and water. These five elements shape up your personality traits and also govern the future course of your life. Everything in nature is made up of these five elements, including the humans. Having an understanding of these five elements is primal before taking up yog or further advancing to the level of kundalini yog.

In *Srimad Bhagavad Gita*, there are volumes on kundalini, outlining the conversation between Lord Krishna and Arjun. Explicitly, these compositions illustrate the behaviour, relevance, significance and the outcomes of kundalini activation.

The entire process of kundalini awakening comprises of several steps and stages of varying energies, defining as to how kundalini would be traversing through various chakras and hollow bones in the spine.

May 2021 **Vishal Dwivedi**

1

Kundalini Power: An Introduction

All the things, including life, have a core in themselves. In life, core is the level of consciousness which a person has. In general, the level of consciousness is based upon experiences—good or bad. The ability to deal with and come out of those experiences is what life is all about. This book is about realising the core of life—the energy which is making you live, think, enact and react. The aim is to realize these energies and find the best alternatives for further growth. In Sanskrit, these confluence points are called *chakras*—"the wheel". It is the very structure of the wheel which makes it unique, as there is no end or a start point. We can also say that the start point is the end point and the end point is the start point. The principles of energy are the same since there is no end to it and neither is there any start.

These energies travel up and down and have swaying movements whilst travelling in the core, much like the movement of a serpent, which drapes on the ground while moving forward. In a similar fashion, these energies drape the spine till the fifth chakra and then take a different shape and movement, which is more semi-spherical. Pertinenly, sages who have mastered the chakras, tend to feel an upward movement when in a deep meditative state.

It has been long realised and found, that in human body, the power resides in the form of emotions and organ driving energies. However, in any of these states, the energy is unstable and keeps varying, while moving towards something else, either a place or a state, which this energy aspires to be in. Later, this state is realised, in which the energy is completely stable and progressive (in Hindu scriptures, namely the *Vedas*, this is illustrated as the *shakti* aspiring to meet

Shiva). In all of humans, at the very onset of their lives, this is the state where it is present and it won't be wrong to mention that this is its primal state. Still, in order to gain more from this invisible power and be able to connect with the other invisible energies of the universe, sages (the people who were aware of the energies) discovered and realised that there are greater chances and possibilities to take these energies to higher levels. Following this realization, further exploration and experiments (including venturing to high altitude areas, like the Himalayas) were adopted to assist in this study.

During the process of self exploration and while ascertaining the path of this/these energies, it was realised that post reaching a certain level, this/these energy(ies) tend to change their behavior, which is also reflected in the way the inhibitor/owning the body perceives the world and other things in the society. This state is known as the state when the *shakti* has reached Shiva, and is considered the most stable.

अश्वस्थमाबलिव्यसोहनुमाँशचविभीषण
कृप: परशुरामश्चसप्तौतचिरजीवन:
स्तौतानय: समरेनित्यमार्कण्डेयमथाषटम्म
जिवेदवर्षशतमसोश्श्शपिसर्वव्याधिविवर्जित

Make no mistake to take this to be the ultimate state, as the real spiritual journey begins now and death shall be conquered, and the energies leaving the body shall not happen and its intensity is so high that nothing is "impossible" for a person.

There are illustrations of what a "kundalini power" can do if and when activated, not only from the spiritual angle/facet but also in the sense of benefits that translate, for attaining greater gains in the societal world too. This illustration has been repeated in many Hindu and Buddhist scriptures. As for example, "kundalini" in yog vashsihta is acknowledged as an emotion, to experience emotions—the sense which provides a sense. रसौवैस: It is a force, which when activated, energises the chakras, and then there is nothing which is impossible for a person—the intellectual and spiritual levels of a person holistically gets "transformed". The perceptions and takes of life emerge completely different to what they were before the pre-kundalini activation. It is a kind of archetypal force which needs to be understood first before one tries activating it.

Kundalini is a Sanskrit word, drawn from snakes, which when sleeps, tends to form a coil and drapes itself on it. Likewise, kundalini is an energy residing in the root chakra area, which is coiled three and half times around the spine, and when activated, goes to the crown chakra and eventually beyond it. It is a master energy of the body, by which the body can see things which aren't visible and know things which are still unknown. The very statement of "tomorrow being uncertain" doesn't hold its veracity with such a realised person; as the person acquires the ability to sense and know what is going to happen.

During the process of activation of kundalini, there is a huge release of energy, and due to this sudden release of energy, the human body is unable to hold onto to its conscious self most of the times. Let me elaborate this by citing a personal experience. I was sitting in a designated posture, completely unaware of things happening around me and remained in that state for several hours; and the same remains even today, while meditating). As a teacher, I have been witness to many a cases, whereby the pupils were in possession of their senses (not completely awakened, but intermittent) and in a state of high energy but without any control over the same. They were not able to channelise that energy for a certain task that they intended, but were rather driven by the power of kundalini. It is not that something nasty or wrong happened with them. They appeared good, but the sense of pleasantness did not co-exist. This scenario is not only with the students but there are many a masters too, who claim to have their kundalini awakened. Altough they may profound, yet, they too are unpleasant and emotionally unstable.

To experience pleasantness when kundalini is awakened depends directly on the natural spectrum of energy with which one is born (the astrological natal chart). This is so because the blessings of the *shakti* can only be had with grace, as there is nothing which can allure her. When kundalini moves up and down the body, in most of the cases, severe pains are experienced or there is a jerking in the body. This also portrays that kundalini is not persistent at all times but is rather intermittent in its virtue. It comes, lays its effect and then coils back, which of course cannot be said to be progressive.

As has been seen with a majority of people, the activation of kundalini is not in their control, meaning thereby that they cannot control its rise and further movement. It is triggered by certain other factors, which is not ideal. This normally happens when kundalini activation happens accidentally (like, while engaging in an emotional event or by drug use).

Kundalini movements are spontaneous, resembling certain *kriya(s)*—just like a wave pattern, which is not stable and rises and falls. Practicing yog postures, reciting mantras (in their correct texture regards frequency and wavelengths), and breathing exercises are best ways to prepare the body for the release of this energy. Noticeably, people are seen more inclined to approach the kundalini at the very onset of it rather than preparing for the system to suit it. Incomplete literature and methodology available on the internet has immensely contributed to people landing in a state of dismay post activation of the kundalini, as none of them encourages the person to adapt and adopt the mandatory tenets.

The living which makes the living possible—in Devi (*shakti*/power) puran, it is mentioned in greater detail which gives all the colours/flavours of life:

1. The power to manifest just by its wish भू
2. The power to perform any and everything, without being engaged into it भुवः

3. The power to know and realise, why of each and everything स्व:

Kundalini, found its name, the "serpentine power", due to its movement within the body, especially during the times when it is just starting to get activated. The forward and swaying movement of the body is more or less its endeavour to compensate for the release of huge amount of energy from the root chakra. This energy travels greater than the speed of light. Post realisation and activation of the kundalini power, four major types of changes or unique powers are exhibited by an individual, namely:

1. वेखरी: The power of speech, which translates into the predictions of such a realised soul and always comes true.
2. परा: The ability to sense and read the thoughts of others.
3. मध्यमा: The ability of speaking what is true. Howsoever insensitive it may seem, but a realised person would only speak what is true.
4. पश्यन्ती: The ability to see the disembodied and travelling energies, and the ability to communicate with them, not by the use of language but by understanding their essence.

नवचक्रंकलाधारमत्रिलक्षयव्योमपंछकमसमयगेतन्नजानतीसयोगीनामधारक:
The one who knows, recognises and respects the existence of nine chakras, their flow, sixteen planks, and the five types of ether, it is he who has realised the energy within...it is he who can claim to be a student of yog.

These nine chakras, which are drawn from the positioning and behaviour of the energy driving chakras, are as follows:

1. ब्रह्मचक्र Brahm Chakra
2. सवादिशठानचक्र Swadishthana Chakra
3. नाभिचक्र Naabhi Chakra
4. हृदयचक्र Hriday Chakra

5. कंठचक्र Kanth Chakra
6. तालूचक्र Taalu Chakra
7. भूचक्र Bhu Chakra
8. निर्वाणचक्र Nirvaan Chakra
9. आकाशचक्र Aakash Chakra

अष्टचक्रनवद्वारदेवनापूर्योध्यातस्याहिरण्मय: कोश:
स्वर्गोंज्योतिषवृत:

Eight chakras and the nine openings in the body when mastered, give the owner the pleasure as it is in heavens

The eight chakras are named as per their behaviour and not as per their positioning. They are, namely:

1. आनंदचक्र Anand Chakra
2. सिद्धिचक्र Sidhi Chakra
3. आरोग्यचक्र Aarogya Chakra
4. कवचचक्र Kavach Chakra
5. सामर्थ्यचक्र Samarthya Chakra
6. सौभाग्यचक्र Saubhagya Chakra
7. संशोशनचक्र Sanshoshan Chakra
8. शापचक्र Shaap Chakra
9. मोहनचक्र Mohan Chakra

Post realisation and activation of this serpentine power, the physical and behavioural personality of a person changes, inculcating and exhibiting a unique and differing kind of aura than the rest of the people around him/her. This persona is not dependent upon the oratory skills of a person, but just the mere presence of a person makes him/her stand different and out of the crowd. A realised person is able to read the thoughts of other people and has the ability to gaze through their energy spectrum and understand the cause of their distress and dismay. The *karmas* of other people are evidently known to the realised soul. If one is able to activate the hidden and unknown kundalini power, the person can then assess the movement of energies in the universe too. Such a person is one with all the other activated energies, popularly known as *devtas* in Hinduism and Buddhism.

यद्ब्रह्माण्डेतत्पिण्डे

The constituents and energies of the body are the same which makes the universe

Upon activation of the kundalini power, a person becomes master of the eight superpowers, namely:

1. अणिमा: Meaning that such a person has the power to increase or reduce the weight as per his/her wish—thereby implying that it can float in air or sink in earth.
2. महिमा: Meaning that such a person can increase or decrease its size as per the wish. This can also be interpreted as, a person not having any definite size.
3. लघिमा: Meaning that such a person is able to heal any infections or diseases by virtue of its own energy.
4. गरिमा: Meaning that such a person's virtues are respected by people who have not even met him/her.
5. इशतव: Meaning that such a person can influence anyone by its aura.
6. वाशित्व: Meaning that such a person, just by the display of thoughts, has the ability to mesmerise anyone.
7. प्राप्ति: Meaning that if a person is desirous of anything (which normally has been the case), it can be had just by wishing for the same.
8. प्राकाम्य: Meaning that a person is respected everywhere; but as per the experience, respect or disrespect has no effect on such a person.

In addition to these energies, such a person is able to sense things which are physically far away and is also able to influence them to a greater extent. In addition to being aware as to what is going to transpire in future for that person, by sensing the changing course of stars and the consequent effects, the individual has won over hunger, thirst and other bodily needs also.

It is not that these energies are not present in human beings, but the presence of all of them in one single person is a rarity. Consequently, when this state is achieved, such a person is said to have attained the "magical powers". The great sage Maharishi Patanjali defines powers that can be achieved by either:

जन्मोषधिमंत्रतप: समाधिजा:सिद्धय:

जनम Birth

औषधि Herbs

मंत्र Mantra

तप Deep meditation

समाधि Wilfuly leaving the body

As per the anatomy of the humans, described in Patanjali, there are two main types of nerves नाड़ी viz. ida ईड़ा which drives the right hemisphere of the brain. Air from the left nostril flows when this nerve नाड़ी is active (in practicality, it is during this time, that the cognitive memory plays a prudent role and a person is engaged in thinking about the incidents which have happened in the past, and depending upon the warmth of the breath, the nature of the thoughts are ascertained—pleasant or unpleasant memories). The second nerve नाड़ी, pingala पिंगला, governs the left hemisphere of the brain and is inhaled or exhaled from the right hand side nostril. When this nerve नाड़ी is active, the individual is contemplating about the future (the coldness in the breath coming from the right side nostril; either it is the aspirations which are there at the fore or the obstacles which would be there to achieve that goal).

These two nerves नाड़ी, ida ईड़ा and pingala पिंगला are responsible for the formulation, behaviour, strengths, and weaknesses of the first five chakras (the confluence points of energies). These five chakras define the scope of a person in society and in the sphere of spirituality, and even how close a person should be in realising and activating the kundalini. If any or all of these five chakras are inflicted, the person would be rigid in his/her perceptions and would believe his/her convictions to be the only truth.

Anyhow, proceeding further, when these nerves नाड़ी are in right order and all the first five chakras have been activated, these two nerves नाड़ी confluence into each other and form a different kind of nerve नाड़ी called sushumna सुषुम्रा, which opens up the path of kundalini to reach the अगना and सहस्रधारा chakras. These two chakras are the opening points for associating and connecting with the cosmos. This is the time when the experiences are not accounted for or recorded, as the soul goes beyond the body (more like what happens in the event of death). However, in this case, it is in a controlled manner and the person is able to bring the soul/energy back into the body as and when is desired.

This सुषुम्रानाड़ी has three constituents, namely, vajra, chitrini and brahmn randr (striking and returning sounds). In fact, these sounds (when activated and realised) are responsible for the ionic body to connect with the cosmic self. This connection is a must for kundalini to start rising from the naadi kand, which is situated just at the tip of the spine.

In *Vedas*, the conduit for the energy to travel is called nerves नाड़ी. They come in varying shapes and sizes and amount to 72,000 in number. It is them, who carry the energy from one chakra to another chakra and finally into the organs. By virtue of their siginificant role in the movement of energies, there are dedicated processes in yog, through which these nerves नाड़ी are kept clean and unblocked. The mechanism of deep breathing, controlled breathing and being breathless, shall be discussed later in the book with due emphasis.

The modes and methods of activating the kundalini power have been kept secret. The popularly accepted and widely known notions are distorted and present incomplete knowledge. However, while sharing the practical experience of the author for activating kundalini, swar स्वर observing and then absorbing the phemes as produced by the right and left hemisphere of the brain, would be comparatively easy for the postures योग.

वंब्रह्माणेनम: मंमहेश्वरएनम: विंविशनवेनम:
हुँफट्सहस्त्रारॐनमोनारायणॐनमोभगवतेवासुदेव:
अंआंइईउऊऋॠऌॡएंऐंओंऔंअंअं:

Recounting my own experience, during the process of activation of the kundalini, it is pivotal that there should be variation in the temperature of the breath while reciting the above swar स्वर phemes. If no variation is observed, it shall have no effect on kundalini. Nevertheless, it would still be capable of healing and curing quite a significant number of diseases, including the psychological ailments.

The great sage Patanjali described various functions and virtues of these confluence points (chakras). They are seven in number (as the spine has seven joints) and have direct impact on the societal life, including education/studies, societal behaviour, aspirations, passion, compassion, level of lively nature, addiction and its nature (like frequency of worshipping), emotional level/quotient, skin colour, thought process, speaking tone, smell of sweat, organ behaviour and health. Additionally, many other trivial and significant aspects of life are also governed and defined by these seven chakras (in the natural course, these seven chakras are not in perfect spectrum, as they vary in strength and composition and probably that is the reason for the existence of diversity in the society—the gap between the rich and the poor). In totality, there are 7 major chakras, 21 minor chakras and 86 micro chakras in a human body. Among the 114 chakras, 112 chakras reside within the body and the other 2, outside the body.

Among the 7 major chakras, 1 is present outside the body, over the head region. Moreover, the 21 minor chakras are distributed all over the body. Head, heart, navel, throat and base of the spine are the five main areas of major chakras. In contrast, the minor chakras are located in our hands, legs, tongue, knee, elbow, clavicles, shoulder, eye, ear and nose. All the chakras are not active at all times. Some are prominent and some are latent.

The first step towards realising and opening the power house kundalini, is to balance the chakras in the body, which balance the glutamate and GABA neuro transmitters in the brain. These two transmitters are opposing by their virtue. Glutamate is the one which generates and creates excitement in the body whereas the GABA transmitter is responsible for stability and peace. Having the right balance of these neuro transmitters would ensure opening up of several unknown energies and virtues. The act and art of balancing these neuro transmitters is accomplished by engaging in physical yoga postures, defined breathing patterns, diet induced systems, and/or by using hippocampus area of the brain (which is called समाधि in Sanskrit).

Financially sound people may encounter different health issues, compared to the not so rich people. This is so because, a certain chakra which is latent in rich people and causing health issues, is active in not so rich people and consequently no health issues. Alternatively, whether a dominating chakra in the rich has made them rich, this disparity in life energies can be understood by studying the variations in the physical and biological structures. There are many people with differing structures and these people get affected in different ways (even if they are under the influence of the same event).

Overall, a human body (irrespective of the size or age) has 114 chakras. 108 of them (including the 7 major ones) are more or less aimed towards the societal life and 6 of them towards the initial path of treading into the spiritual world. In the book, we shall be focusing on the popular seven chakras only. These 7 chakras are elaborated and discussed below.

1. Root Chakra मूलधाराचक्र

This chakra is where the kundalini power resides and is responsible for how life would transpire and efforts would translate into. The activation and strength of this chakra make a person an achiever or a dreamer.

2. Solar Plexus मणिपुरचक्र

This chakra is responsible for the fire element in the body and has 10 varying sounds नाद. These sounds, when identified in the right spectrum and strength, helps a person take the right decisions at an appropriate time (as it is not only the right decision which defines success, rather the timing is equally important).

3. Sacral Chakra स्वाधिष्ठानचक्र

This chakra is the controlling point of the water element in the body and has 7 sounds नाद. While germinating and governing the water element, this chakra defines emotions and the emotional strength. Weakness in this chakra can cause several psychological ailments, deformities in blood, addiction to drugs, low esteem etc.

4. Heart Chakra अनाहत: चक्र

This chakra is responsible for the emotional quotient output and has 12 varying sounds नाद. When the energies in this chakra are at the optimum level, a person is judicious in pursuing his/her aspirations and desires. Concurrently, if the energies aren't balanced, a person is always slogging and is under constant stress.

5. Throat Chakra विशुद्धिचक्र

This chakra is responsible for the kind of personality a person would possess and has 23 varying sounds नाद. How impressive and impactful would a person be is defined by this chakra. This chakra is wrongly portrayed as something to do with the tone and sound of a person. Contrarily, this chakra is the first confluence point where सुषुम्नानाड़ी starts its journey towards the higher energy dimensions. This is point where the "me" gets diluted and the "self" starts emerging.

6. Third Eye Chakra आज्ञाचक्र

This chakra is responsible for the concentration and concentrating intensity which a person holds. Self-talking and hallucinations are the common attributes which occur following the imbalances in this chakra. This chakra when activated and being at optimum level provides the possibilities to read the "unsaid" thoughts of other people. This chakra also imparts the scope for time travel and governs the ether element. It is in this chakra, that सुषुम्नानाड़ी disassociates itself completely from ईड़ा and पिंगला with a consequent positive effect of no swaying of the body during the ध्यानयोग.

7. Crown Chakra सहस्त्रधाराचक्र

This chakra is the doorway to the cosmos. It is upon activation of this chakra, that a person shall be able to sense the circumventing and travelling energies. Upon activation of this chakra, a person is able to change the aura and the energies of the other person and is able to visualise things in multiple dimensions.

All human beings have a distinctive dominating chakra. For example, a child has a dominating root chakra which is skeptic to each and everyone. A person who has a dominating sacral chakra is an artist and the one who has a dominating solar plexus is generous and diligent by its nature. The ones who have a dominating heart chakra, are inclined to music, theatre, and/or sculpting. People who can associate themselves with either of the traits mentioned, but aren't following the guiding principles of these chakras, are most likely to suffer from diseases corresponding to these chakras. To explain, a person who has a dominating heart chakra but isn't following the principles of that chakra is more than likely to have a heart ailment. The one who has a dominating solar plexus but isn't observing the associated principles, is likely to suffer with insulin secretion issues and the psychological health of that person is likely to be compromised.

Chakra, undoubtedly, is an energy centre. It is also a centre which coordinates the flow of energy within the body, thereby transmitting the energy to various organs and other confluence points—the other chakras. It receives, assimilates and transmits the energy—the life force—to reach a point where you are able to go beyond the body and its other peripherals. The unblocking of the chakras is very important, rather it is paramount. We can metaphorically illustrate chakras as the various facets of life viz. household, profession, wealth, health, etc. and acting on all of these needs to be in correct order and proportion to enjoy the bliss of "happiness".

The role of each chakra is important and its activation is equally significant too. If any of the chakras is in a latent state, not only the prospects associated with that chakra get influenced, but in totality, there would be an imbalance in life. As previously cited, the gap between the rich and the poor is not because the poor do not have the opportunities to turn rich but perhaps they may not be approaching the things in the right fashion—harnessing the desired energies.

The balancing of the chakras has to be done in a manner in which a chakra is able to perform all the three important aspects, namely, receiving, assimilation and expressing. If any of these aspects is missing, there shall be no resultant advantage or gain. Adhering to the chakra balancing regime requires an in-depth study on the part of teacher to understand which amongst the three aspects of the chakra is lacking.

Correct analysis of the chakra is equally important for healing the chakra. The kind of healing process is also dependent on the aspect which needs to be fixed. An incorrect approach and analysis on the part of teacher can leave a student in lurch without the desired results (unfortunately, there aren't many a masters of chakra yog who are profound enough to deduce a correct analysis).

Like for example, if a person is not able to compensate fully for the energy drawn from the body and replenish it back into the system, the root chakra would be considered weak. These people would have less patience and would possess a high anxiety quotient. Under such circumstances, it is the duty of the teacher to understand the energy spectrum of the student by either talking to him/her (if the teacher lacks the ability to evaluate the energy spectrum by gazing in the eyes or at the forehead) or engaging the student to perform breath holding or muscles stretching exercises.

People in general, without noticing or recognising the chakras, start avoiding things which are a result of some deficient chakra. For example, a person with a deficient heart chakra would not feel comfortable in the company of others or would be harsh in the choice of words, just because of the simple reason that a heart chakra has some or other kinds of sacragges, and there has been no defined process to heal them. Consequently, this avoidance or repulsive attitude develops.

An unbalanced chakra influences other chakras too, making the rest of the journey in yog more difficult for adoption. The problem of one chakra is not limited to that chakra only rather, it is shared with all the other chakras. As mentioned before, a chakra works on three aspects viz. receiving, assimilation and transmission. Therefore, if the receiving is afflicted, the assimilation of the same would also be inaccurate. Subsequently, the transmission aspect of the incorrect assimilation would also impact the working of the other chakra. Like, excessive thinking not only results in hypertension or migraine, it also affects the digestive system of a person and the sequential low endurance of a person.

Hence, for a chakra to be in its correct order, the chakra needs to be balanced and their grounding has to be perfect, as the energy within the chakra is also a kind of electrical energy which needs to be aligned with a potential difference for the current to flow. For the chakra to be able to heal itself there can be various paths which one may choose to tread.

These could range from yog postures, to recitation of the mantras, to breathing exercises or to focus-based exercises. Which one would be best suitable or compatible with your energies should be discussed diligently with your teacher, who would then analyse and suggest accordingly.

It is pivotal to mention here that when the third eye and the crown chakras get activated, a person looses all the inherent fears and there is an impeccable sense of peace in randomness. There is an evident transformation in the behaviour and nature of a person. The person is more than likely to be less emotional or emotion driven and the body thins out, as the ether element replaces the water element in the desired ratio.

The chakras map onto levels that are evident internally as well as externally, and by virtue, they are archetypal energies connecting the inner elements with the existing ones. It is similar to like, the earth on which we walk, the air that we breathe, the water that we drink, and the essence of space/ether that we have within which enables us to feel/experience the outside sphere.

Basically, the chakras are portals between the inner and the outer world. These portals are a conduit to associate ourselves with the elements and their balancing within, for kundalini to awaken.

Kundalini power is the ultimate power which can be attained by virtue of yog; as all other powers post realisation of kundalini, cannot be achieved by performing yog. The powers travel across a person on their own as kundalini establishes a bridge between the cosmic and the ionic energy.

Chakra Name	Location	Element	Virtue	Self	Weakness	Strength	When Weak
Root Chakra	Base of Spine	Earth	Survival	Stability; Grounding; Health; Solidity	Fear	Heavy	Ungrounded; Fearful
Sacral Chakra	2 Fingers	Water	Sexuality	Fluidity	Guilt	Indulgent	Joyless
Solar Plexus	Navel	Fire	Power and Will	Energy	Shame	Dominating; Anxious	Poor Self-esteem
Heart Chakra	Heart	Air	Love	Radiance	Grief	Narcisstic	Shy
Throat Chakra	Throat	Hymns	Associate	Creative	Lies	Loud	Fear of Speaking
Third Eye	Glabella	Light	Intution	Insight	Illusion	Delusional	Poor Memory
Crown Chakra	Skull	Consciousness	Awareness	Union	Attachment	Spiritual	Cynic

Post realisation of kundalini, a person goes into deep meditation and the sense of the senses is non-existent. This also means that whatsoever experiences are in attendance in that deep meditative state, are not recorded or cannot be narrated, as there is no memory of them. That is why, I have opined that no regime is available for acquiring additional powers, post activation of kundalini, since "my" has now taken the back seat and "self" is driving down the things. Self, which can also be reckoned as "soul" or आत्मा, does not associate itself with sensory or memory aspects.

There are eight stages of yog which a person goes through while emabarking on the journey aimed at activation of kundalini. These eight stages are, namely:

1. यम

In this stage, a person divorces all the ill feelings and prejudices.

2. नियम

In this stage, a person modifies the eating habits. Chewing is continued till the time the food is almost in a liquid state before swallowing. A person objectively eats freshly cooked food and only when hungry, and not by the time clock.

3. आसान

In this stage, a person cleanses the prevailing 72,000 nadi नाड़ी by undertaking dhyanyog ध्यानयोग़ breathing execises. The breathing pattern of a person changes, with breath getting softer and easy.

4. प्राणायाम

In this stage, a person practices control over breath, with both inhaling and exhaling mannerisms, witnessing a change.

5. प्रत्याहार

In this stage, a person learns mantras and the correct procedures/principles for their recitation. The recitation of the mantras help in activatating several pockets and parts of the brain, which further strengthen and activates other organs of the body.

6. धारणा

In this stage, the worldly desires and attractions are divorced and the ability of concentration is enhanced and improved.

7. ध्यान

In this stage, the virtue of being away from senses and memory is practiced and mastered to the levels that one is able to sense/see the same in its own self from the outside. This is also popularly known as out of body experience.

Kundalini is draped around the sushumna nadi सुषुम्नानाड़ी in the upper spine area, near to the cervical. Since sushumna nadi सुषुम्नानाड़ी plays no role in day to day life affairs, in a majority of people, it remains in a latent state all its life. The same is true with kundalini too. This is so because, humans in general live with a notion that it is their efforts which would lead them to success or achievements and while upholding this thought process, they tend to forget that it is the inner and other circumventing and influencing energies which are instrumental in materilization of things. Resultantly, the quest for finding/realising these energies does not exist and eventually the "life transforming" energies remain in a latent state.

पश्चिमाभिमुखयोनिगुद-मेढ्रानतरालगा!
तत्रकन्दसमाख्याततत्रासतेकुंडलिनीसदा! सामवेशटासक्लानाड़ीसा ्ध्र-त्रि-
कूटीलाकृति:! मुखेनिवेशयसापुचछ: सुशुमणा-विन्नेस्तिथता!!

Nadi नाड़ी and chakras are deeply related with the four forms of life energies viz., physical energy, mental energy, emotional energy and the spiritual energy. For an ideal life, there is a need to balance these four energies. These four forms of life energies are interrelated and overlap each other. Chakras play an integral role in balancing these four energies and keeping our mind and body healthy. When balanced, our chakras strenthen the immune system and enhance body's ability to heal itself.

There are numerous nadis नाड़ी and chakras present in our body. However, 72,000 nadis नाड़ी and 114 chakras are the most prominent. Unlike machines, life energy moves up and down in a rhythmic fashion. The energy flow in the नाड़ी is linked to the sleep cycle—the circadian rhythm and the ultradian rhythm of the body. Ultradian rhythm is associated with the sleep cycle, hormonal secretion cycle, brain wave frequency cycle, blood flow cycle, and brain hemisphere or lobe dominance cycles. Normally, the duration of ultradian rhythm cycle is about 90-120 minutes.

This ultradian rhythm of the body is maintained by the 72,000 nadis नाड़ी of the body. These 72,000 nadis नाड़ी are densely connected with the navel area, heart area and the brain area of the body. Nadis नाड़ी are a part of our astral as well as the causal body. They are the channels and fields of life energy and consciousness. The network of nadis नाड़ी can be classified into three groups, namely, the collection point, the purification facility, and the distribution network. Collection points are directly associated with our six senses. The distribution centres are mostly associated with our glands and the mid-brain. They collect, store, filter and prioritise the incoming information and energy. Finally, they send the refined information and energy to the purification facilities. The distribution points include the junction points on the surface of the body. They are at the intersections of different muscular patterns, joints, tendons, ligaments, bones, arteries, veins, nerves and subtle energy points.

As outlined in saraswati rahasyopanishad सरस्वतीरहस्योपनिषद, the fingers of the hand are the terminals of elements. The little finger कनिष्ठा represents element earth, the index finger अनामिका represents water, the middle finger मध्यमा represents the ether/sky/space element, the ring finger तर्जनी

represents the air element and thumb अँगूष्ट represents the fire element. These elements not only play a meangiful role in the spiritual world, but are also critcal for day to day activities. It ranges from the choice of food to the amount and quality of sleep desired. The choice to read a book is also attributable to the dominating ether element, which encourages you to know thyself beyond the body.

As is well-know, a human body is made up of five elements, namely:

1. Fire अग्नि: Governs your sleep, the quality of sleep, passion towards things and life, aspirations and hunger for food, and laziness.
2. Ether आकाश: Governs emotions of life viz. guilt, remorse, compassion, anger, dismay, and addiction.
3. Air वायू: Governs speech, tone, ability to forgive and forget, and sulking.
4. Earth पृथ्वी: Governs stability, being grounded, and cynicism.
5. Water जल: Governs the intensity of emotions, colour of your skin, heart and the mental health.

These five elements shape up your personality traits and also govern the future course of your life. Everything in nature is made up of these five elements, including the humans. Having an understanding of these five elements is primal before taking up yog or further advancing to the level of kundalini yog. Each of these elements represents a state of matter. Earth is not just soil, but is basically everything which has a shape and size. Water is everything which is liquid, either flowing in the form of water, or present in a sedimented form as ice or in a vaporous form. Air is everything that is gaseous, may it be without any water content. Fire is a part of nature which is able to change the existing form of an element, for example, changing water into air. That is the reason why fire is worshipped in all the religions. In Vedic system, the procedures to change the course of the things—destiny—is also done with the help of fire. It is popularly known as "tantra" तंत्र. This tantra तंत्र is of two types, namely, vaam margiy वाममार्गिय—the one which is performed using the phemes, and dakshin margiy दक्षिणमार्गिय—the one which is carried out using the commodities (flora or fauna).

Element space is believed to be the mother of all elements. It is in this element that all the other elements pour in. In its natural course, the percentage share hovers around 3, but following the process of kundalini activation, the value jumps to 30 percent. During the course of deep meditation, it is this element which provides "space" for the soul to remain preserved and yet travel.

A strong interrelationship exists amongst each of these elements and their association varies from person to person. There has hardly been a case where all these elements have been at their optimum level in the natural course. Some of the elements, by virtue of their existence in a person, are contradictory and cancelling in nature. For example, if the composition of fire and water is not in correct proportion, it can prove destructive for each other.

If the ratio of water element is high comparable to the fire element, it may lead to inflammation in the body, heart ailments, and different types of cancer, as a resultof this imbalance. Contrastingly, if the fire element dominates over the water element, a person may likely suffer from Parkinsons, Alzheimers, muscle dystrophy, intestinal malfunction or liver cirrhosis, and renal lesions/failures, consequent of this imbalance.

Each element has a unique role in contributing towards formation and working of the body. Element earth is instrumental in providing shape and size to the body and to the organs in addition to determining a prescribed smell, structure of the skeleton, muscles, skin, tissues and hair. Water element is responsible for carrying out the excretory functions.

Formation of saliva, urine, semen, blood, sweat, and lubrication of blood vessels are some of the tasks discharged by element water. Element fire is responsible for catalyzing hunger, digestion, thirst, sleep, flawlessness in skin, avoiding blood coagulatation, hair colour, and nail formations to keep the body in a dynamic state. Element space provides clearance from illusions and delusions, as it forms attraction (both in physical and the spiritual world).

If any of these elements are imbalanced or their confluence is not corresponding with each other, the likelihood of ailments—physical, biological, or psychological—intensifies, and if this imbalance is left unanswered or unattended to, it may culminate in failure of organ(s).

In human body, water is expressed in five distinct ways, popularly known as the *kapha*. The water that protects mouth against the actions of chewing and the enzyme that assists in breakdown of carbohydrates (salivary amylase) is called bodhaka kapha बोधककफ़.

Bodhaka kapha is a salivary fluid, present in the mucous membrane secretions of lips, cheeks, and pharynx. Water that protects the mucous membranes of our stomach against acids that aid in digestion is called kledaka kapha कलेदककफ़. The water that stabilises the flow of neurological impulses and protects nerves of the brain is called tarpaka kapha तरपककफ़.

Water that protects joints from the friction of motion is called sleshaka kapha सलेसककफ़. Sleshaka kapha सलेसककफ़ is found in the synovial fluid that moistens joint surfaces, and in the bursae that allows tendons to glide smoothly over each other.

Water that protects the respiratory system from the movement of breath (a drying process) is called avalambaka kapha अवलंबककफ़. Avalambaka kapha अवलंबककफ़ keeps the mucous membranes of the bronchi and lungs healthy and also provides fluids that support the pleura and pericardium.

Water and the Kapha Dosha

The kapha dosha contains both water and earth. It is the water that is responsible for most of the protective and healing aspects of kapha dosha. As water is the foundation for earth in the body, an increase in the water characteristics would result in weight gain and sluggishness.

Consequences of Excess and Deficient Water on Dhatu धातू

Tending of water in the body begins with caring of kledaka kapha कलेदककफ़ in the stomach. The stomach is home to kapha dosha. If an upswing in the quality of water is witnessed, it results in an overflow from the stomach onto circulation and consequent flooding of tissues in the body. If the food ingested is too moist or oily, water builds up and reduces the strength of the digestive system. Subsequently, digestion becomes impaired and the food moves slowly through the digestive system.

The accompanying loss of appetite and a sense of heaviness in the abdomen are among the early signs of an increase in kapha, indicating its imbalanced nature. As water overflows from the digestive system, it often settles in the watery tissues of the body. These tissues are, namely, the rasa रासा (plasma), meda मेधा (fat), shukra शुक्र (fluidic reproductive tissue) and dhatu धातू.

The increase in quantum of these tissues results in edema, obesity, and enhacement in genital waste secretions (smegma). Concurrently, the secondary watery tissues also surge, resulting in an increase in menstrual flow and breast milk supply in women. Unfortunately, the quality of the increased breast milk and menstrual fluids is poor and often mixed with mucous.

Pertinently, water deficiency has scores of fallouts. The rasa रासा, medha मेधा and shukra शुक्र become too dry, resulting in dehydration, dryness of mucous membranes, dry skin, weight loss, and weakness in reproductive tissues. A dry rasa

रासा also results in decrease in urination, sweating, and the formation of dry hard stools. In addition, the lips and eyes too become dry.

Water in Diet

While examining the dietary structure, it would be worthwhile to mention that sweet taste is the main source of water. Cooked grains, non-fermented dairy products, nuts, and fatty meats are examples of food having ample water element. Proper and adequate intake of these food products supports a healthy mix of water element in the body. However, excessive intake would result in symptoms aforementioned and an inadequate intake would lead to symptoms of deficiency.

Element Fire

The element fire, called agni अग्नि in Sanskrit, is the third of the five greatest elements (pancha mahabhutas पंचमहाभूत). It is placed third since it evolves from ether and air, containing the essence of these elements within. Ether provides fire the space to exist within, while air provides fire the capacity to burn. It is because of air that fire is never still. Fire element represents the capacity for heat and light. Fire is a generator of energy in the body just like sun is a generator of energy for the planet earth. Fire represents all sources of energy in the world including solar, hydroelectric, nuclear, fossil fuel and bio-diesel. Fire is a process of liberating energy from its source.

The origin of element fire vests in the tanmatra तन्मात्रा of vision called rup रूप. Rup रूप means form or colour and both are a result of perception.

Rup रूप is the tanmatra तन्मात्रा, or primordial, un-manifested form of perception, light, and vision. Fire and visual sense share a special relationship. Fire provides light for perception. The eyes are a vehicle through which light is digested and perception takes place. Hence, disorders of visual perception are primarily correlated to element fire.

Feet are an organ of action closely associated with the fire element. Using feet as a medium, we react to what we see. By putting into operation, feet allow a person to change the course of direction based upon perception. Not only can the direction be changed, but also the intensity of progress. The choice of direction and the intensity of action are ethos of element fire.

In order to understand an element, it is importat to be aware of its attributes. Fire is hot, luminous, dry, rough, subtle, flowing, sharp, clear and soft. Fire is neither stable nor mobile. Fire neither stands still nor generates motion. Inherent within the fire is air, and it is this air that equips fire with its mobile aspect. Although fire is subtle, its effects are clearly visible, generating a clear sense of its nature. It is the heat of the fire that is most recognisable.

During the ancient times, the idea of fire was quite comprehensive for the sages. Fire represents light, heat, lustre, energy, understanding, metabolism, and the power of transformation. In human body, fire is expressed in five distinct ways. Fire that provides our body with the capacity to digest food is called pachaka agni पाचकअग्नि. The fire that ignites the intellect, digests ideas, and allows for understanding is known as sadhaka agni साधकअग्नि. The fire of perception that that digests visual impression into recognisable images is called alaokik agni आलोकिकअग्नि. The fire that energizes and invigorates the body, adding color to the body is called rajak agni राजकअग्नि. The fire that digests touch and sunlight and gives off the radiance associated with healthy skin is the light provided by bhrajaka agni भराजकअग्नि.

Because of the destructive nature of fire, it is always blended with a small amount of water in the body to prevent any harm to the tissues. The repository of fire and water is known as *pitta*. Hence, the five variants of agni अग्नि are also denoted as five types of pitta.

Overabundance of fire in the body results in the buildup of heat, and a deficient proportion could spark symptoms of cold. There are also other ramifications of heat. As it builds up in the body, there is a need to eliminate the excess heat. Resultantly, the body sweats and urinates more, and the stools become loose and frequent. The lustre of skin increases and the eyes shine brighter. The mind becomes sharper and more focused while the intellect strengthens. If the fire increases in quantum, there are negative consequences. There is eruption of skin accompanied by red rashes; eyes become bloodhot, intensity of mind increases; tissues of the body may suffer from inflamation, and there is likelihood of fever. Contrarily, lack of fire in the body results in skin losing its lustre and turning grey or pale with a consequent slow down in metabolism. The repercussions are also felt in the digestive system with improper digestion of food. Mentally, it becomes taxing for the mind to digest new information. As the body tries to hold on to heat, sweating, urination, and bowel movements decrease.

The pitta dosha contains both fire and water but it is the fire which plays a dominating role. Hence, any vitiation of fire will ultimately result in vitiation of pitta. Pitta remains healthy as long as fire in the body is well tended.

Tending of fire in the body begins with monitoring of pachaka agni पाचकअग्नि or the fire of digestion. When digestive fire is healthy, there is little gas and elimination occurs on a regular basis (almost 1-2 times per day). Digestive fire is aggravated primarily following the consumption of hot, spicy, and salty foods. Comparatively, it diminishes when there is an intake of heavy and cold food. Hence, if the digestion is weak and the fire is low, the dietary mix should be made lighter and spicier until the digestion normalises.

The whole creation is made up of five elements, blended in different proportions. In our diet, pungent, sour, and salty tastes embody maximum fire. Out of the above, the pungent taste would escalate fire most rapidly. However, it is the sour taste that has the long-term effects. Pickled food, yogurt, and foodstuffs marinated in vinaigrette are examples of sour food.

Summer is the season of fire. During this time of the year, the rotation of earth around the sun results in longer daylight hours. Naturally, summer is the most active time of the year. As long as the weather does not become unbearably hot and humid, summer is the time to carry out things planned/deferred during winters and the spring time. It is the time of the year to work diligently to fulfil *dharma*. However, there is a need to be watchful, for if a person becomes too focused and intense, the magnitude of fire will intensify and pitta will become vitiated. Thus, it is important to keep the proportion of fire in check while maintaining a diet that is cooler and less spicy.

While perceiving the cycle of life and death, the quotient of fire symbolizes the extent of most productive years. If one is well prepared for this cycle of life during one's youth, these years purposed for the fulfilment of dharma. An individual's capacity to work is maximal in this phase of life. Regardless of the constitution, while monitoring the transition from puberty till the old age, the penetration of fire is prominent in all the human beings. For those, blessed with a fiery nature, it burns the brightest and these individuals must be cautious not to commit themselves to the extreme and burn out.

Element Earth

In Sanskrit language, human body is referred to as "parthiv" पार्थिव/पृथ्वी, meaning that the entire structure of the body is based upon element earth. May it be bones, muscles, hairs, nails, ligaments, tendons etc., all are associated with the element earth. Tarka Sangrah illustrates element earth further, as anything and everything which contains a smell or can generate smell that is "earthly" in nature; it is called गंधतत्व. There are two types of element earth, namely:

(a) Nitya Prithvi नित्यपृथ्वी: This connotes the eternal component of earth. It is small in proportion, but is supposed to be the creation of functional and effective earth.
(b) Anitya Prithvi: This comprises of the non-eternal component, derived from the eternal component. This part of element earth is "naturally" effective and activated, but for the root chakra to be activated, nitya prithvi नित्यपृथ्वी needs to be stimulated and extended a dominant role.

Earth is basically of two type viz.: (i) eternal and inconsistent, and (ii) microscopic and invisible. The role of element earth is so vital that it has been linked even with the formation of foetus. The building up of the form, its stability, and the holding of foetus as a single mass is associated with element earth. Element earth provides solidity to a structure, without which a body cannot be modelled and would collapse if formed. Element earth utilizes water element in building up bones, muscles etc. and provides a definite shape and size to it. The consumption of raw earth by some pregnant ladies is also an indication of the lack of element earth in their body.

The very occurence of faeces is also related to element earth. Of course, in faeces, there is element water too, but without element earth, the body won't be able to cleanse itself. Same goes for urine too, as any deficiency of element earth in the body would result in pungent smell emanating from urine and there would also be an uncontrolled flow in urine passage, as what is witnessed during the renal malfunctioning and/or failure. The relative balance of element earth with other elements is equally significant. As expressed in Ayurveda, when this element is present in a balanced proportion, the possibility of lesions or damage to internal or external organs in the body are minimal. This element provides shape, colour, and odour to all the organs.

If element earth is unbalanced—either independently or in combination with other elements—the following ailments are most likely to occur:
1. Weak and/or brittle bones

2. Osteomalacia
3. Osteoporosis
4. Pathological dislocations and ligament tears.
5. Osteopenia
6. Osteoarthritis
7. Renal calculi
8. Atherosclerosis
9. Tooth fall or additional tooth/teeth
10. Constipation
11. Persistent pain in legs and pelvis area
12. Low HB count

In addition to this, there is a persistent anxiety and remorse within a person who has a deficient ratio of earth element. If element earth is disturbed and on the excessive side, disorders like stones in kidney, urinary bladder, and atherosclerotic plaque in the blood vessels, could be anticipated. In not so rare cases, thinning of the blood vessels to alarming levels has also been witnessed.

If there is an imbalance in other elements in addition to element earth (which is commonly seen), systemic diseases like gigantism, acromegaly, obesity, hardening of the muscles, including those of the internal organs, also transpire. When element earth is relatively low in proportionality, commonly occurring diseases like baldness, skin decolouration, acne formations, black spots on the skin, polio, asthma, bronchitis, and allergies happen.

Imbalance of element earth can be attributed to many reasons. Amongst them, the most common relates to the kind of food and the mood in which we consume the same. The speed of consumption of food, time taken to ingest and digest food, stale or packed food, unnatural and processed food etc. are some of the other determinants.

Element Air

Air is called vaayu वायू in the Sanskrit language, and evolves from the ether element which has varying potentials embodied in itself, resulting in the formation of air. It is dynamic in nature, thereby possessing the possibility and provisions to change its value at any given point of time because of the kinetic energy factor. In normal course, it remains stable in value, and can only be altered by attempting a specific bandha बंध. It assists more or less in the movement of energies to and from the chakras. This process can be hampered if any variance is observed in the chakras which will consequently affect element air.

Sparsh स्पर्श is the potential of a touch experience, expressed in the most subtle form. Basis the trait that touch and air are inseparable, skin is correlated with element air, as it is through skin that we can touch or feel. Skin has typical characteristics of being mobile, cool, dry, rough, sublte, flowing, sharp, clear, and hard. Although air is subtle, the effects are quite significant to sense the same. Element air is associated with our breath. Consequently, it is one of the most important elements for survival.

Any imbalance in this element could be corollary to premature mortality, compared to disproportion in other elements. Element air is responsible for pran प्राण. Sages have described element air as possesing five forms, keeping into consideration the criteria of movement. These five forms are:

1. Apaan अपान
2. Vyaan व्यान
3. Udaan उदान
4. Samaan समान
5. Pran प्राण

In body, element air is expressed as a form of motion and corresponding life. It provides energy for the flow and circulation of blood within the body, nerves to impulse, and neurones to mitigate and travel.

When element air is in excessive proportion within the body, hyper excitability is experienced whereas a deficient proportion would result in dullness.

Element Ether

Ether is known as aakash आकाश and can be implied as a space which all other elements occupy. It can also be presumed as completeness, in "hollowness". Ear and mouth are the organs broadly associated with this element, and any ailments related to hearing or speech can be correlated with disequilibrium in element ether. Ether draws all its virtue in contradiction to other elements. Probably, that is the reason, it is able to accommodate all the things, including the other elements.

Ether is the one which encompasses the possibility of blending with any or all other elements, without changing their essence. However, it is the behaviour of other elements which is altered during the chakra yog; in order to retain their behaviour and results in control. Brain is the organ associated with this element. The importance of brain cannot be undermined by the sheer fact that the functioning of body is conclusively dependent on brain and the scope extended by element ether for its balancing is very minimal, because of its virtue, simplicity and complexity. There are traces of element ether in other organs also including blood vessels, intestines, bladder and lungs. The hollowness in the bones, especially in the spine, also has traces of ether, becaue of which there are greater sensations in the spinal area when there is an upward movement of kundalini.

Illustrative Representation of Aasana

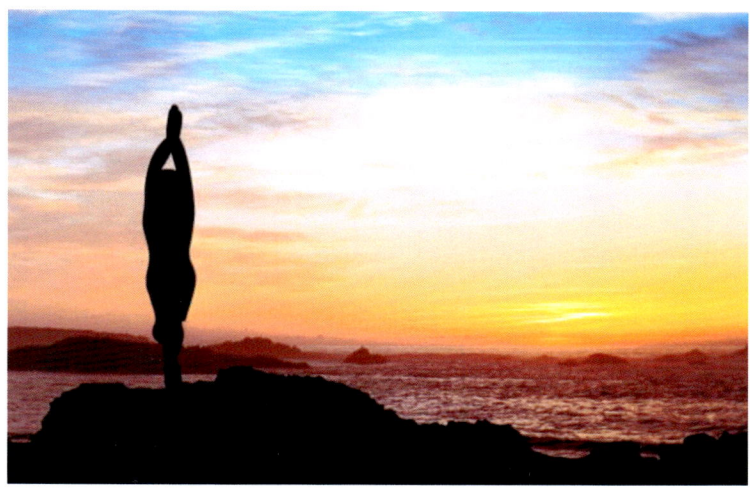

Illustration: Chakra Mudra चक्र मुद्रा

2

Root Chakra: Mooldhara

There are seven major chakras (confluence points) in the body which are responsible for the energies to travel upward and downward. These seven chakras are the seven major joints in the spine; the spine that hosts the three nadis नाड़ी, clearing and activation of which is the key to unblocking the hidden energies within. As elaborated in the introduction to the kundalini power, there are numerous methods enshrined in the *Vedas* and several others, which have been developed by the sages during their journey of realization. These include:

1. Breathing स्वाँस
2. Physical योग
3. Hand Formulations बंध
4. Focus-based Exercises ध्यानक्रिया
5. Mantras Recitation मंत्रउच्चारण
6. Naad Kriya धुनीयोग
7. Yantra Sadhna यंत्रसाधना
8. Tantra Sadhna तंत्रसाधना

In the chapters on chakras, I shall be illustrating various techniques specific to all of these chakras, and how and what shall be the initial sensations or experiences that one may encounter while undertaking them. The later experiences may vary from individual to individual and presenting a generic experience as to what one should feel, post crossing the first benchmark of unblocking these chakras, would be wrong on my part. However, I would definitely highlight the hallucinations which one may undergo, post the activation, in order to circumvent one's way and not get stuck in the same.

In this chapter, I will explain the first chakra, mooldhara मूलधारा. As the name suggests itself, this is the inception point of the energy to implore and explore. This chakra when activated pullulates in four directions viz. North, South, East and West. The sages who observed the movement of the chakra have illustrated this luxuriation in the yantra यंत्र which is a pictorial representation of the movement of energy in the chakra. The four directional movement of the energy in this chakra also represents society and has great value pertaining to gains in the societal life. This chakra or the first 5 chakras when stimulated and activated, extend prosperity in both the worlds—societal and spiritual. The exclusive spiritual journey starts post crossing the throat chakra. It is then, when the aatman आत्मन stretches out to parmatmam परमातम्म and the gains in the sense of wealth, fame, name and other frills of life aren't really desired and the person really doesn't languish to have them either. Anyhow, I shall continue to share the procedures and techniques to activate these 5 chakras.

Three positions and the ellipsoid—the four directions are reflection of what kundalini is and her behaviour and how she would move (if and when that is the case). Kundalini is just an opening of the tail bone (the lowest part of the spine). It is this opening which hosts the mouth and the tail of kundalini even when it is in a latent state. With the onset of the regime of opening of this chakra, the kundalini starts its movement (this depends upon the existing energy spectrum and the balance status of the elements).

Self-control, known as Indra इंद्र, is the power of activating this chakra. As per the purana पुराण, इंद्र rides brown coloured elephant with seven trunks and each of these details has their relevance in understanding and hence activating the chakra. The brown colour of the elephant indicates the colour of the organ/area where this chakra is (when blood is washed, this area is brown in its colour). The seven trunks of the elephant reflect the way this chakra interacts and communicates. The names and virtues of these seven trunks are:

1) Shrot श्रोत

2) Twacha त्वचा
3) Chakshu चक्षु
4) Jivah जिवाह्
5) Naasika नासिका
6) Guda गुदा
7) Ling or yoni लिंगयायोनि

These seven virtues of the trunk are responsible for all the seven colours and seven notes of the music and also how the seven major planets would be for an individual.

The reason for reflecting "elephant" as the vehicle वाहन of इंद्र "self-control" is that since times immemorial, humans like elephants, have always been languishing for more than what they can consume. Having utmost sincerity towards the "self-generated" needs and desires, there is no end to the consumption and it often destructs those/that who are not even blocking it. However, the one who has mastered his/her desires, lust and greed, is the one who shall be riding this uncontrolled elephant (which possesses immense power and energy, but just needs the direction and the right path) and making the best out of this energy. This is what the yantra यंत्र of this chakra means.

The mantras as mentioned in yog vashisht योगवशिष्ट associate Lord Ganesha as the epicentre of this chakra. In the mantra recitation process of activating the chakras, it is the beej mantras बीजमंत्र of Lord Ganesha which are recited. Of course, there are definite and prescribed principles as to how the recitation should be done.

The reason for associating Lord Ganesha as the epicentre of this chakra is derived from the four directional movements; as is the case with Lord Ganesha who has four arms, and in these four arms, Lord Ganesha is depicted as holding:
1) Modak मोदक: symbol of joy and jubilation
2) Kamal कमल: symbol of prosperity
3) Ankush अंकुश: symbol of control(ing)
4) Abhay Mudra अभयमुद्रा: to be fearless

The northern junction (looking upwards) of the triangle is associated with Lord Brahma ब्रह्मा, as it is at this junction, where exists a possibility of the energy from this chakra to take four new forms/purposes, viz.:
1) Bhautik Sharir भौतिकशरीर: worldly pleasures
2) Baudhik Sharir बौधिकशरीर: intellect
3) Bhavnatmak Sharir भावनात्मकशरीर: emotional
4) Chaitnyatmak Sharir त्मकशरीरचेतनया: consciousness

Bhautik Sharir भौतिकशरीर: This virtue of life and the facet of human body is the one which takes care of or generates the need for worldly pleasures like hunger, sleep, emotions, liking or disliking and all other traits which are conceived to be societal or existential.

Baudhik Sharir बौधिकशरीर: This virtue of life and the facet of human body is the one which generates emotions post the "evaluations" of a thing or an event. The corresponding emotions of success or failure driven post the thing are absorbed and observed by this part of the body.

Bhavnatmak Sharir भावनात्मकशरीर: This virtue of life and the facet of human body generate "love" and "prejudices". The deductions in the Bhaudik Sharir बौधिकशरीर are complied and analysed and resultantly, the corresponding emotion(s) pertaining to "love", "acceptance", "prejudice" and "defiance" are released.

Chaitanyatmak Sharir चेतनयात्मकशरीर: This virtue of life and the facet of human body are responsible for recognising and absorbing "knowledge" or "learning". Academic performance is also governed by this facet of human body.

Any person when behaves in a selfish manner and doesn't adhere to the axioms of nature, it is then when the person inflicts this chakra and the results are detrimental. There may not be immediate visible effects but sooner than later, issues pertaining to health, profession and personal life are "enhanced".

As mentioned above, there are three ways by which chakras can be stimulated and regular following of (any of) these measures will ensure opening and hence the activation of the chakra. Before I mention the ways which you may adopt for activating the chakras, I shall be enlisting food articles at the end of each chapter which shall assist you in activating the respective chakra.

Breathing

Breath is one of the most difficult thing to alter and also keeping it in a specific manner, as both biological and psychological facets of the body shall be dithering post this change.

For the stimulation of root chakra, you need to sit in sidh aasan सिद्धआसन.

The breath needs to be inhaled both from the nose and the mouth. In the event of inhaling air from the mouth, the intake should resemble as if you are eating something and it has be swallowed (like drinking water), pushing the air from your lungs to the lowest part of your posture. When you are able to make the breath reach the lowest part of the body, hold it there and keep you cheeks in the manner of "mouthful" duration for holding the breath within. This will depend on your personal capacity and shall increase with regular practice (mentioning any time period would contribute to stress building as the aspirants would be focusing more on the timeline instead of the breath, which is what I do not intend to prescribe).

Keep repeating this exercise for at least half an hour in one sitting and doing twice a day would help a great deal. Importantly, there should be a gap of at least 3 hours between the exercises and the food consumed. In addition to the minutiae of the exercises, the ambience would also contribute towards the success factor. Room temperature set at 22 degrees would be beneficial during the initial days as also sitting on a blood coloured mat (preferably having the yantra of root chakra inscribed on it) would assist in your endeavour of activating the root chakra.

Physical Postures

The tenets of this part of the regime are based upon the releasing and blocking/restricting the flow of blood and other nutrients to specific parts of the body. In yog, for root chakra, a person has to sit in sidh aasan सिद्धआसन.

While being in sidh aasan सिद्धआसन and before starting yog, one should do deep breathing exercises in which the breath has to be taken more than in the "regular" fashion and has to be held in the chest area (time period for which the breath is to be held in the chest shall depend upon your lung capacity, but effort should be made to increase the breath holding period) and released as slowly as possible to ensure that all of it is exhaled before you inhale afresh. Repeat this breathing and relaxing/warming up exercise for 10-15 minutes, before moving on to physical yog.

While being in sidh aasan सिद्धआसन and ensuring not to move your lower torso, bend forward while exhaling and try and touch your nose to the ground in frontal position. Hold this position whilst not breathing till the time you are comfortable. Under no circumstances, you should try and be uncomfortable with any of the exercise(s). Even if you are unable to carry out the postures or the breathing at the very onset, do not worry, as it shall come with regular practice, post holding yourself in front stretched position.

Subsequently, bend backwards while inhaling (the level of bending shall depend on your flexibility) and hold the position till you can balance yourself without using the hands. The next step is to bring yourself back to normal sidh aasan position and take breathe normally to relax yourself, before repeating the exercise. Repeating at least 20 times in one instance would be a good number to start with and then you may choose to increase the frequency. If you have problems doing sidh aasan (which is a clear reflection of blocked root chakra), you may do the exercise keeping your legs stretched forward initially. However, do work upon gathering the flexibility for doing sidh aasan.

(Refer to Illustration 2.1: Sidh Aasan सिद्धआसन *at Page No. 47)*

The following aasan's are not the standalone ones compared to the one mentioned before. They all need to be done in the order as being presented.

Apanaasan अपानआसन

As you are aware, the root chakra is at the tip of the spine. This aasan आसन helps in stimulating the tip and the corresponding muscles of the area. Lie down on your back with your legs extended forward, and slowly bend your knees one by one or at one go, depending on the existing strength of the pelvis area (at no point of time, stretch yourself beyond your comfortable limits) and move these bent knees towards the chest area. You will experience the lifting of the tip and of the spine too. It is okay if it rises above the ground but do try to keep it to the ground while moving your bent knees towards the chest. When your knees have come close to the chest, grope them with your arms and hold them while keeping your breathing normal.

Release the position and gently place your feet on the ground in forward extended position and relax and keep your head and rest of the body on the floor. Now, slightly lift your legs, hold them and then release. At this point, you should be feeling some sensation in the tip of the spine. In case you are not that observant, you can feel the change in the muscles surrounding the spine.

(Refer to Illustration 2.2: **Apanaasan** अपानआसन *at Page No. 47)*

Ardh Hal Aasan अर्द्धहलआसन

Lift your legs straight without bending the knees and try and bring them together over your head. Hold it there for the duration as long as possible while maintaining normal breathing or close to normal. Under no circumstances, you should hold the position if you are feeling breathless or an extra effort is required for breathing.

Now, bring down both the legs at a very slow pace, and while coming down, try and hold on to each of the position for sometime before coming down further. It must be ensured that you are using your front abdominal muscles and the pelvis muscles. At no instance, you should hold it if your back is not relaxed and is bending upwards.

Post the feet touching the ground, relax for a little while before attempting another set of this exercise. Reduce the resting period on your way as you build up your muscles.

(Refer to Illustration 2.3: **Ardh Hal Aasan** अर्धहलआसन *at Page No. 48)*

Supta Padangusthasan सुप्तपदंगुस्तआसन

In this aasan आसन, the inner muscles of the legs and the bridge joining the legs are stimulated, which helps in activating the root chakra.

Spread your arms completely at shoulder height and then lift your leg and try and touch the hand of that side while rotating your head in the opposite direction. Repeat the same exercise on other side also, whilst ensuring that there is no stress on the back and there is a feeling of stimulations on the "bridge" of the legs.

(Refer to Illustration 2.4: **Supta Padangusthasan** सुप्तपदंगुस्तआसन *at Page No. 48)*

Setu Bandha Sarvangaasan सेतुबंधसर्वांगआसन

In this aasan आसन, you need to lie down on your back, with legs stretched forward. Now, bend your knees and lift your pelvis while keeping your shoulders and head on the ground. Hold onto this position and bring your arms in the space created by lifting up of your lower torso and let the hands clip together.

Hold this position for as long as possible, and when you choose to return, first untangle the hands and move your arms to the side of the body and gently let your body touch the ground. As your torso has touched the ground slowly, stretch your legs forward and relax before repeating the exercise.

(Refer to Illustration 2.5: **Setu Bandha Sarvangaasan** सेतुबंधसर्वांगआसन *at Page No. 49)*

Salbhasna Aasan सलभसंआसन

In this aasan आसन, lie down on your belly with arms close to your body and palms facing the ground. While keeping your head straight and on the ground, lift your leg straight upwards and hold it as long as you can comfortably. At no point, should you exert yourself and bend the leg. Now, bring your leg down and let it softly touch the ground. Repeat the same process with your second leg too while adhering to all the requisites.

(Refer to Illustration 2.6: **Salbhasna Aasan** सलभसंआसन *at Page No. 49)*

Bhujang Aasan भुजंगआसन

In this aasan आसन, while lying down on your belly, bring your folded arms close to your chest and by using the strength of your arms with support of the spine muscles, lift your upper torso from the ground while keeping your pelvis and lower torso on the ground.

Now, lift your body and stretch backwards while keeping the maximum weight on the arms, which would be almost straight by now. Hold on to this position at your comforting levels and then slowly return to lying on the belly position.

(Refer to Illustration 2.7: **Bhujang Aasan** भुजंगआसन *at Page No. 50)*

Aadh Mukhas Aasan आधमुख्बासआसन

In this aasan आसन, lie down on your belly with your arms around the chest area. Now, lift your pelvis area by bending backwards from the lying position. Keeping lifting your pelvis area till the time your arms and legs are full stretched. Hold onto this position till you are in your comforting limits.

Now return back to the initial stage and rest for a while before repeating this exercise again.

(Refer to Illustration 2.8: **Aadh Mukhas Aasan** आधमुख्बासआसन *at Page No. 50)*

Uttaasan उत्तासआसन

In this aasan आसन, stand straight on an even floor and lift your arms stretched over your head and very slowly bring them down, touching the back of your heels (you may stick to touching the ground during the initial days and when you acquire flexibility, you can touch the back of the heels). Hold the position while keeping your breath normal. Now, release the aasan and bring back your body to the standing straight position. Relax for sometime before repeating the exercise again.

(Refer to Illustration 2.9: **Uttaasan** उत्तासआसन *at Page No. 51)*

Ardh Hanuma Aasan अर्धहनुमाआसन

In this aasan आसन, sit in a posture with knees bent but upper legs in an erect position. From this position, stretch one of your legs in front of you and with your arms touching the ground, try and sit on the leg which is bent. Now, try and touch your nose with the knee of the stretched leg. Hold this position for as long as you can comfortably and maintain it while breathing normally.

Hereafter, bring back the stretched leg to the bent position and repeat the exercise with the second leg. It is important that the duration of holding remains the same for both the legs.

(Refer to Illustration 2.10: **Ardh Hanuma Aasan** अर्धहनुमाआसन *at Page No. 51)*

Supt Viraasan सुप्तवीरआसन

In this aasan आसन, you have to be in a kneeling position with feet comfortably apart from each other. Now, try and sit back in between the feet and hold this position for a while. While holding the body in between your legs, bend your back backwards so that you can lie on your back while keeping the knees bent. Hold this position for as long as you are comfortable while maintaining normal breath.

From this point forward, slowly (without any jerks) lift your back and come to the kneeling position and get up standing straight on your legs. Relax for a while before repeating the exercise.

(Refer to Illustration 2.11: **Supt Viraasan** सुप्तवीरआसन *at Page No. 52)*

Hand Formulations

The fingers of the hand are joined in a specific manner to facilitate the stimulation of specific chakras. This exercise is called bandha बंध. The tips or the roots of the fingers are the areas where the same nerves or corresponding nerves travel, which are positioned there or affect the chakras. In the case of root chakra, join the tips of your thumb and your index finger, (kindly ensure that there is no pressure of pressing on either the thumb or the index finger) called the sidh mudra, and inhale hard and keep inhaling as per your comfort zone. Hold the breath in your lungs and push the entire held up breath to your belly and then gently and slowly breathe it out (the amount of time taken to exhale should be at least double the time taken to inhale). Keep repeating this exercise for at least half an hour before normalising your breathing patterns.

(Refer to Illustration 2.12: **Hand Formulations** *at Page No. 52)*

Focus-based Exercises

This is one of the most difficult facets of the exercise (as per the response received from students and clients). This is so because it requires keeping your mind quiet and focusing on something which is a part of you (as till now mind has been focusing on things other than the body). The pre-requisites include sitting in sidh aasan and observing sidh mudra सिद्धमुद्रा formed in your hands, comfortably resting on the folded knees. Thereafter, take your focus to the tip of the tail of your spine and keep it there and use your psychological powers to stimulate the tip. It is quite similar to what is done while tickling. Hold onto your position for a significant period (just beyond your comfort levels, as they would be), release the focus and come back and open your eyes. Take a gap of few breaths before restarting the above mentioned exercise.

Mantra Recitation

The confluence point (root chakra) while undertaking either of the following: (a) receiving, or (b) assimilating, or (c) transferring, generates a sound which is recoiling in nature. Simply putting, it engages both the inhaling and the exhaling part. The pheme of this chakra is "LAM", and while reciting, kindly ensure that you are reciting all the three letters of the mantra. For the benefit of the readers, it is suggested if they can adopt the following procedure for reciting the mantra:

LLLLLALALALAAAAAAMAMAMAMAMMMMMM

Naad Kriya

This is the most prominent stage of chakra meditation. In this stage, the sound, as produced by the mantra, is heard from within the body and during the hearing process, the reactions of the brain are also observed which correspond in accordance with the chakra producing the sound. For you to be able to adopt this process, you should be very comfortable. Without any break, while undertaking focus-based meditation for more than a couple of hours, there would exist a possibility of you being able to reach the inner self to the extent of realising the motions and hearing the sound.

Yantra Sadhna

This yantra of root chakra is formed by formulating the body (using hands, arms and legs) in such a way that when you breathe, the stimulations caused by the usual posture of the body are caused at the root chakra. For the root chakra, twist your legs in such a way that they entangle/grope each other while standing and then repeat the same for the arms too with a difference that at the end of the groping of the arms, the palms of the hands should face each other.

Hold onto this position while breathing normally till the time you are comfortable, and then gently entangle your arms and legs. Thereafter, relax by engaging in normal stretching exercises and repeat it again. It is recommended that your holding period while following this formulation should be at least 20 minutes (total of the repetitions) initially and later on, you may choose to increase it as per your strength and endurance.

Tantra Sadhna
This facet of the chakra meditation is beyond the ambit of this book.

Illustrative Representation of Aasana's

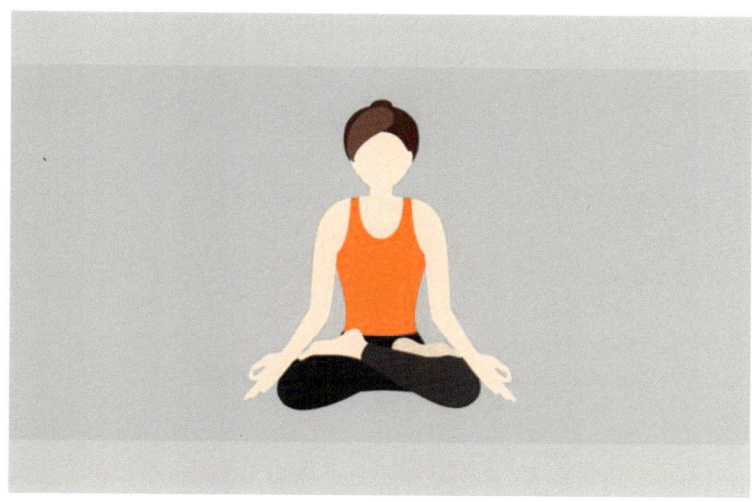

Illustration 2.1: Sidh Aasan आसनसिद्ध

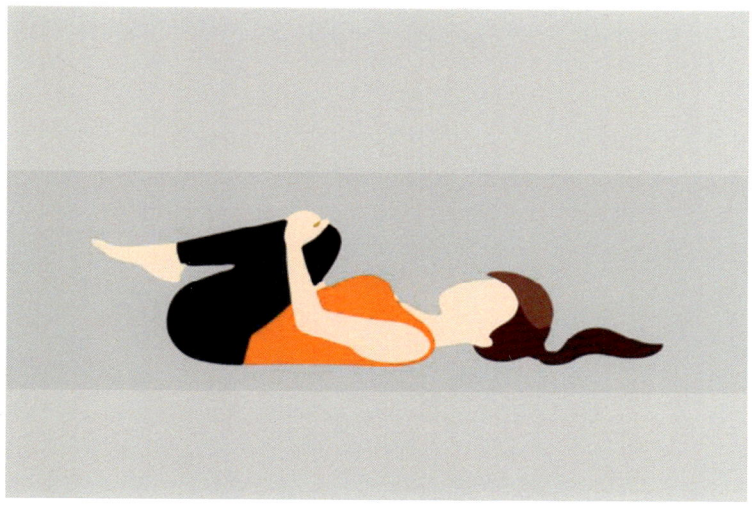

Illustration 2.2: Apanaasan अपानआसन

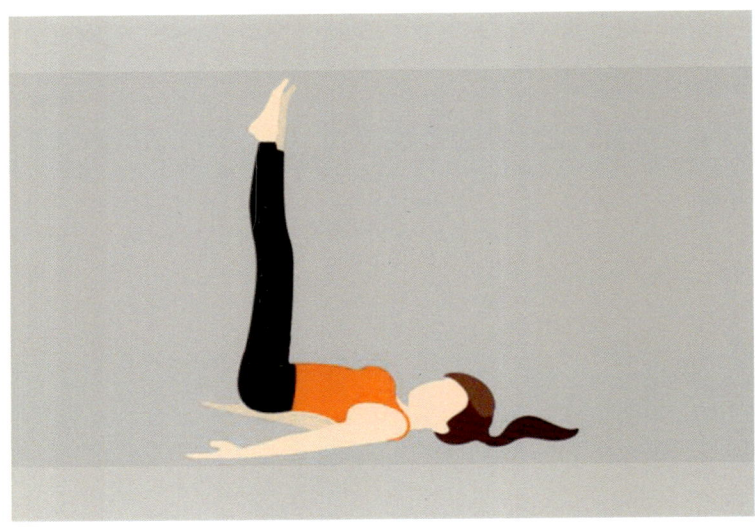

Illustration 2.3: **Ardh Hal Aasan** अर्धहलआसन

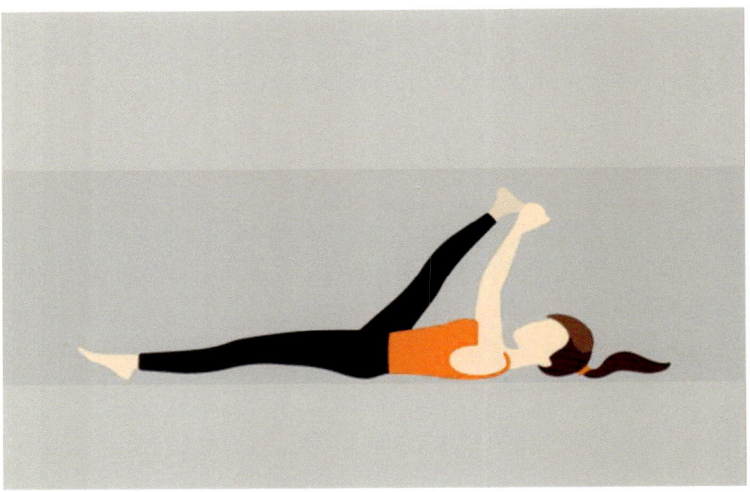

Illustration 2.4: **Supta Padangusthasan** सुसपदंगुस्तआसन

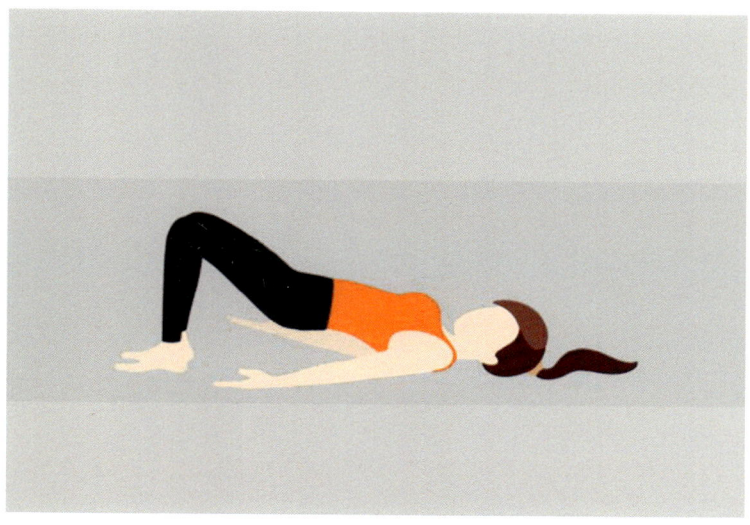

Illustration 2.5: Setu Bandha Sarvangaasan सेतुबंधसर्वांगआसन

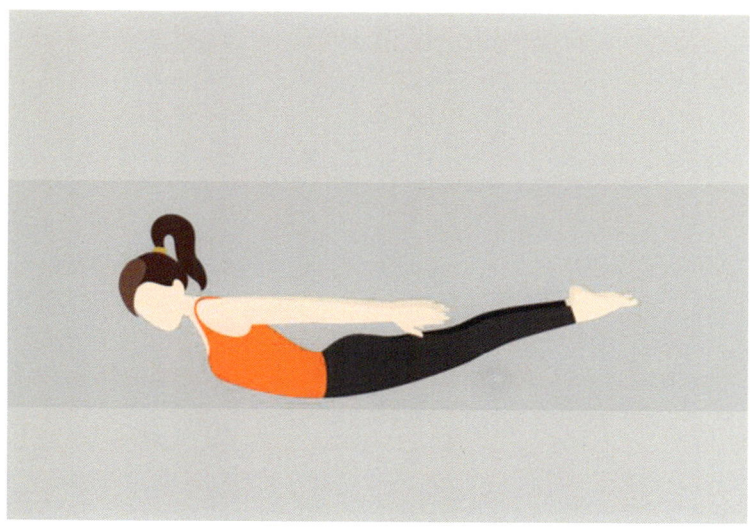

Illustration 2.6: Salbhasna Aasan सलभसंआसन

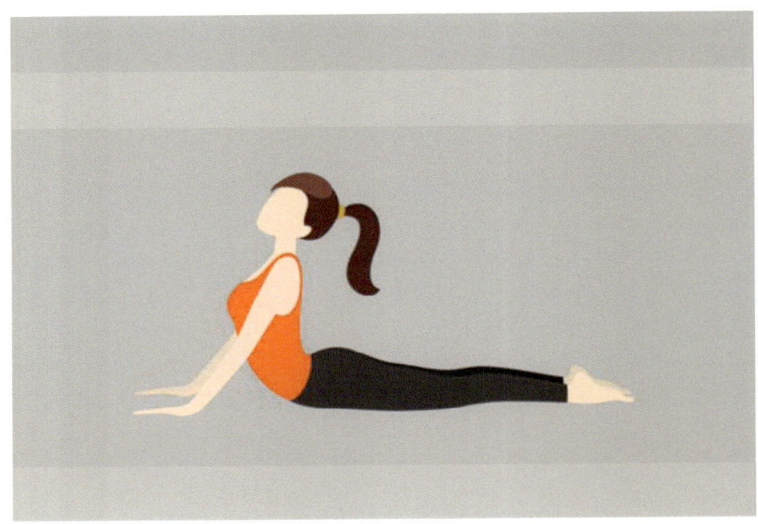

Illustration 2.7: Bhujang Aasan भुजंगआसन

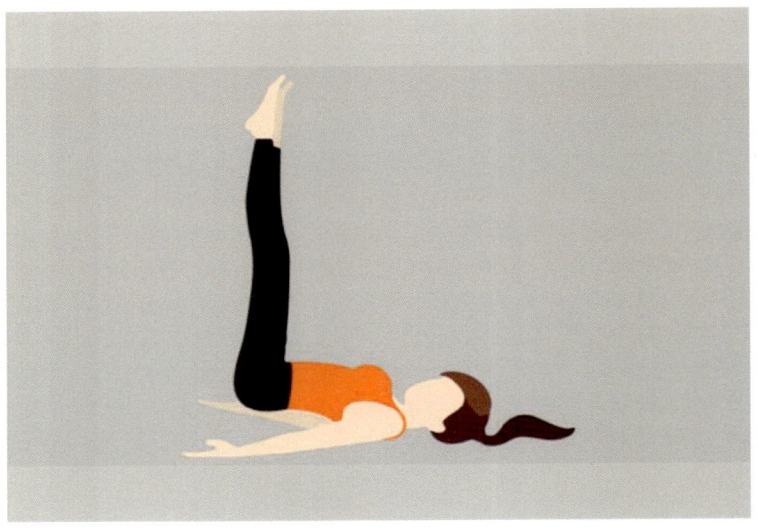

Illustration 2.8: Aadh Mukhas Aasan आधमुख्रासआसन

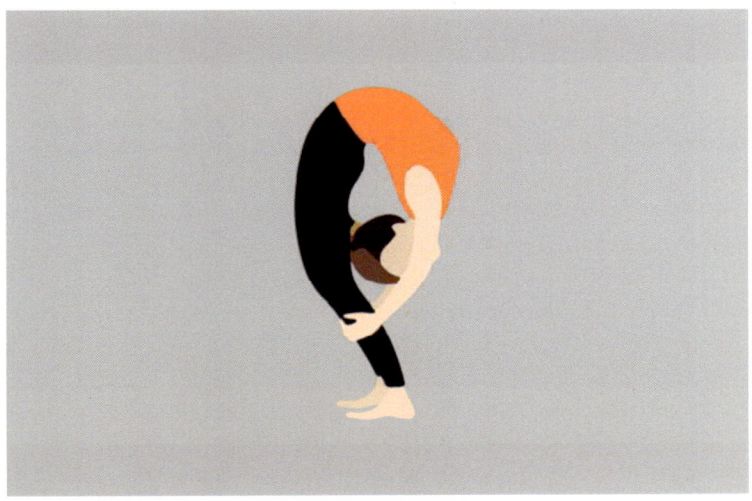

Illustration 2.9: Uttaasan उत्तासआसन

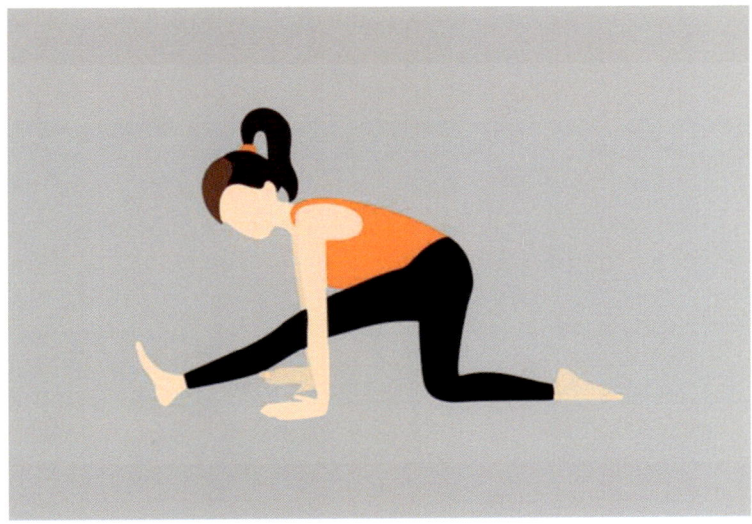

Illustration 2.10: Ardh Hanuma Aasan अर्धहनुमाआसन

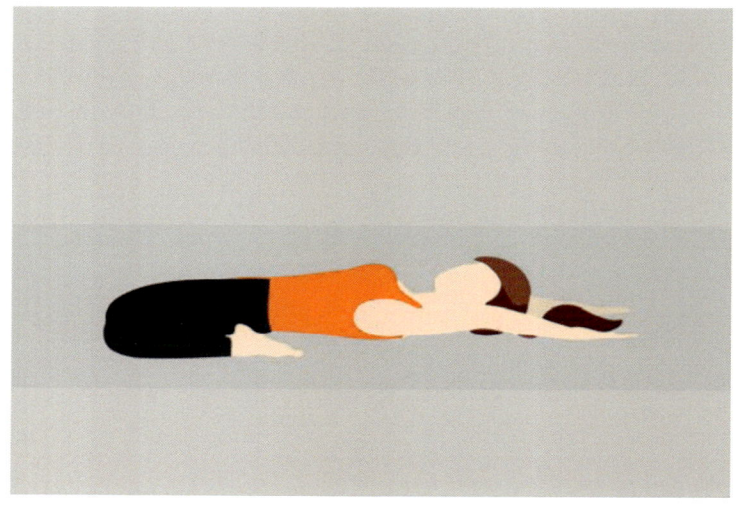

Illustration 2.11: Supt Viraasan सुप्तवीरआसन

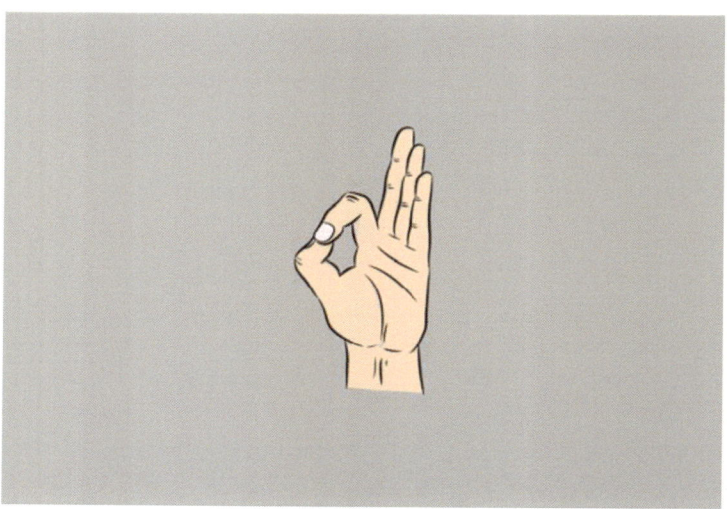

Illustration 2.12: Hand Formulations

3

Manipura Chakra: Confluence of Fire, Water, Air and Earth Elements

This chakra in Sanskrit language is called manipura chakra मणिपुरचक्र and in English language, it is referred as the Solar Plexus. Irrespective of the language it translates into or the point of origin, it is this chakra, from where the energy starts manifesting itself in various forms and these forms can be engaged to get the desired results. Irrespective of what the texture of work may be, these energies when activated can lead to accomplishment of anything. If not, there would be struggle in each and everything in your life, right from the basic requirements to the more advanced needs. This chakra is responsible for valour and courage. Comparably, it can also be stated that this chakra is responsible for the confidence in oneself and its abilities to accomplish the things.

A person who has activated manipura chakra lacks no confidence to undertake a task. The ability to accept and then learn is a perfect example of "valour and courage". Located above the navel, manipura is translated from the Sanskrit language, meaning the "city of jewels" and is also alternatively translated as "resplendent gem" or "lustrous gem". Manipura is often associated with the colours, namely, yellow, blue in classical tantra, and red in the Nath tradition.

Manipura is associated with fire and power of transformation. It is said to govern digestion and metabolism, as it is home to *agni* and the vital wind *samaa vayu*. The energies of *prana vayu* and *apana vayu* (inward and outward flowing energy) meet at the point in a balanced system.

Manipura is the home of coeliac plexus, which innervates most of the digestive system. In chakra-based medicine, practitioners work in this area to promote healthier digestion, and elimination of impurities in pancreas and kidney for improved adrenal function. Weak agni (fire) in the coeliac plexus leads to imperfect digestion of food, thoughts and emotions, and is a source of *ama* (toxicity).

तनमध्येसिित्रिनीस: प्राणवविलसितायोगिनमयोग़मायालुतातनपमेय:
सकल:सर्जिनम: मेरुमध्यातराअशठानमभित्वडेडिप्यातेतड-ग्रथन:रसायनसुधा-
बोध:-स्वरूपा-तनमध्येब्रह्मनाड़ीहरमुख:-देवन्नत्रआत्मा

For the sake of understanding the above Sanskrit verse, which illustrates the positions, functioning, relevance and significance of this manipura chakra, here is a broad translation.

"Inside her is *citrini*, who is lustrous with the lustre of the *pranava* and attainable in yoga by yogis. She (citrini) is subtle as a spider's thread, and pierces through the lotuses which are placed within the backbone, and is pure intelligence. She (citrini) is beautiful by the reason of these lotuses which are strung on her. Inside her (citrini) is the *brahmanadi*, which extends from the orifice of the month of *hara* to the place beyond, where Adi-deva is".

Manipura is represented with a downward-pointing red triangle, signifying the *tattva* of fire, within a bright yellow circle, with 10 dark-blue or black petals like heavily laden rain clouds.

The fire region is represented by the god Vahni, who is shining red, has four arms, and holds a rosary and a spear. Vahni is making the gestures of granting boons, or favours, and dispelling fear. He is seated on a *ram*, the animal that represents Manipura. Agni is referenced later as well, as Hinduism altered over a period of time. Fire is the dominant element in this chakra, but as described in the title itself, this chakra is the confluence point of fire, water, air and earth. This is so because, anything and everything to have a shape, needs at least these four elements. Of course, the importance and contribution of ether and space can never be discounted, for that shape to be relevant and significant. This chakra apart from the inward energies is dependent on the vision for its functioning. The sense of butterflies in the stomach upon witnessing something which isn't anticipated can be taken as an example to understand the relevance of vision for defining the functioning of this chakra.

This chakra receives and transmits energy into ten different channels, each one of which has its own phonemes, which is also reflected by the various assimilations occurring in this chakra. Shunya mudra शून्यमुद्रा is a mudra which is formed in the hand. While focusing on this chakra, the entire emphasis should be on two things, viz. the energy travelling post the formulation of the mudra and the effect it is generating in the chakra. One should be able to observe the desired changes, and if the changes are not visible, an express methodology should be applied to realise it. This is so because engaging in any exercise without its recognition is a "total waste" of time and energy.

Manipura is considered the center of dynamism, energy, will power इच्छाशक्ती, and achievement, which radiates *prana* throughout the entire human body. It is associated with the power of fire and digestion, as well as with the sense of sight and the action of movement. While meditating on manipura, one is assumed to attain the power to save, change or destroy the world. The position of manipura is stated as being behind the navel. Sometimes, a secondary chakra called *surya* (sun) chakra is located at the solar plexus, whose role is to absorb and assimilate prana from the sun. Being related to the sense of sight, it is associated with the eyes, and being allied with the movement, it is associated with the feet.

In the endocrine system, manipura is said to be associated with pancreas and outer adrenal glands (the adrenal cortex). These glands create important hormones which are beneficial for digestion converting food into energy for the body, just like the way manipura radiates prana throughout the body.

The very basic understanding of the levels of activation or blockage of this chakra can be evaluated from the receptiveness of the taste buds in tongue and/or by the formulation of saliva, whether it is thick, normal, less or more. You must have noticed that some people even spit while speaking. This is a reflection of dysfunctional manipura chakra, as when problems of digestion exist there is a sense of confusion—discernibly, there is a change in the way saliva is formed in the mouth. The cleanliness of tongue is also attributed to the functioning of this chakra. If this chakra is activated, there shall be no bad odour in the mouth and the tongue would bear a light pink colour. People try achieving this in a cosmetic way also, but in the natural course, if manipura chakra is activated, the mouth would be free from germs and any bad smell. Interestingly, the person would be observant even for minute variations in taste thereby suggesting the sensitivity of taste buds.

The second organ to observe and monitor, to understand the strength of the manipura chakra, is by evaluating the normalcy in vision. Concerns like, a person having weak eyes, formation of slush in the eyes, dryness in tear glands, redness in the eyes, sleep related problems, and characteristics of dreams, could be assessed by understanding the behaviour of this chakra. Primarily, the above outlined discomforts would make a pitch for a definite prognosis by a teacher/guru to suggest a suitable method/technique to be adopted for the activation of manipura chakra. As there is no rule of "one size fits all" in chakra, yog and/or kundalini yog, it is by the wisdom and experience of a teacher/guru, that you shall be able to achieve the desired result.

When manipura chakra is out of alignment, digestive issues arise. This could be evident in the form of improper processing of nutrients, constipation, or irritable bowel syndrome. Eating disorders, ulcers, diabetes, issues with the pancreas, liver, and colon are some of the symptoms of imbalance in this energy center of manipura chakra. An imbalance can also cause severe emotional problems. It can start with doubt and mistrust towards people in your life, and continue in the form of worrisome behavior about people's perception about yourself. Some people may even experience low levels of self-esteem, resultantly searching for continuous confirmation and approval from others. This imbalance may lead to unhealthy attachments with people in your life. Activating manipura chakra cultivates a willingness to gain insights into the understanding of power, individuality, and identity. In some people, a misaligned solar plexus chakra can make skilful self-expressions challenging. In others, it may be manifest as overly rigid, displaying a controlling behaviour. Also, it may breed a victim's mentality, neediness, and lack of direction or self-esteem to stand up and take recourse to a positive action.

As mentioned above, in manipura chakra, there are ten main nerves which blend (and also impact in a standalone mode), which as per dakshin maargiy दक्षिणमार्गिय, is a reflection of ten main forces शक्तीरूप. These main forces शक्तीरूप are responsible for ten most crucial facets of your life, namely:
1. Worldly
2. Societal
3. Family
4. Wealth
5. Health
6. Children
7. Profession
8. Fame and Recognition
9. Intellect and Education
10. Personality and Smartness

All the above listed dimensions could be augmented if one is able to stimulate and activate the manipura chakra. Although, it may sound too simplistic to be true, yet never discount the fact that what you are, what you think, and what you do, is all because of these energies, and in case you would like to improve upon the things, change the nature/behaviour at source and the result would be visible in itself. The ten kinds of energies which are influenced by this manipura chakra include:

1. Praan प्राण
2. Aapaan आपान
3. Smaan समान
4. Udaan उदान
5. Vyaas व्यास
6. Krum क्रूम
7. Dhananjay धनंजय
8. Prtaksh प्त्क्श
9. Aprtaksh अप्त्क्श
10. Sukshm सूक्ष्म

Also, there are seven major types of unformulated energies which emerge out of this chakra. These energies then take the shape of infinite number of things/formations which accordingly define life and the results obtained thereupon. These seven forms are named as:

1. Kaali काली
2. Kraali कराली
3. Manoliva मनोलिवा
4. Sulochita सूलचिता
5. Dhumvarna धूम्रवरन
6. Safulingini सफुलगिनी
7. Vishavruchi विश्वरुचि

As described earlier, fire is the most dominating element in this chakra, and for fire to be there, there needs to be a correct amount of friction and space. If there is friction and there is no space, there shall be no fire and if there is too much space, the amount of fire generated would be trivial. In yog and more so in chakra yog and kundalini yog, physical body is just to assist in the stimulations, supposed to be done subtly. It is this energy body, where all the life energies dwell and behave from. The chakras are the confluence points of these energies. We can envisage them as battery banks, which need to be charged so that they can release the chakra. In chakra yog, this is what is achieved. We charge these chakras, which can be used as and when the need arises. Fire is the dominant element of the manipura chakra. However, there are additional elements attached to this element. For any of the other element/s to engage in a role or establish significance on to the energy body, the fire element needs to be regulated for both the generation and the release. It won't be wrong to assume this to be the innuendo of the regimes associated with the manipura chakra. One can feel the rise of this heat within when one engages in physical yog, mantra recitation, or naad kriya. If no such experience is felt, I would urge you to check and take corrective measures.

As described above, valour and courage are the most dominating virtues which arises post activation of this chakra. There is no discounting the fact that these two virtues would be in dire need even when you would want to activate this chakra or as a matter of fact any chakra, so as to induce the body do what it is trying to resist and keep repeating it time and again. For this to materialize, you have to have a strong zest for the thing, or else you would be inclined to enhance your energies beyond their present state. There are few species, including floor and fauna, which have the provision of regulating the heat within. We humans are not one of them. However, the variations that we see around or terminology like "dysfunctional" is because it is not conventional on our part to have lower levels of heat than the natural benchmark. And yes, there is no doubt when this chakra is activated, you can increase or decrease the fire element, post having control over it, but that would require a certain and specific expertise. To achieve this, the component of mastery is of paramount importance. Undoubtedly, it is not a time-based thing. It can happen much sooner than you would anticipate or may not happen at all. What amongst these would hold true with you would depend on your approach and a diligent analysis by your teacher/*guru*. Which element is more assisting and which is repulsive and how the repulsive one can be circumvented, would be subject to the activation of manipura chakra of your teacher/guru which in turn would facilitate his/her sensing of your energies and subsequently suggesting a suitable path that would be most productive and less time consuming for yourself.

When manipura chakra is in a healthy alignment, it eliminates insecurity. This leads to recognition of inherent power and the feeling of empowerment. Connecting with a strong purpose in life enhances a deeper understanding of the individual contributions while measuring success. This brings prosperity in personal and professional life. Letting go of negative things becomes easier since dependency on others is reduced. There is a marked improvement in recognising self-worth rather than focusing on material things. This positive transformation is brought about by consistent practice to investigate and identify the symptoms of blockage. A well-balanced solar plexus chakra enables us to effectively plan and achieve success. Cleaning and opening this chakra can transform a person into a better leader and create an inspiring life by repeating positive affirmations about personal power. Through repeated affirmations, either by asserting out loud, or in our heads, or by writing them down, we help reverse negative thought patterns and replace them with the constructive ones.

Your focus, manifestation, ambition, and paramount virtues of fear and/or gain are derived from the solar plexus. When we are out of balance here, we may face control issues, hypersensitivity, action imbalances, and issues with our health in the form of anxiety and blockages in digestive system. Fear and augmentation of negative responses prevent us from moving beyond the built up negative space and rather than keeping us safe, they prohibit us from healing in our desire, thought and fear. Solar plexus is the source from where people receive the incoming energies.

Breathing is a phenomenon of discharging emotions in tense situations. The tool combines the power of heart and gut to enable you to shift emotion and physiology right in the middle of a strong reaction. Record and write down irrelevant and non-conclusive thoughts you may have and more positive attitudes you wish to have. Guide yourself with alternative perspectives you think could help. For example, while pursuing a nemesis in our life that redirects the flow of our objectivity, we can choose breath—breath love, breath appreciation, breath compassion or breath excitement—and experience the same. Following the experience, you shall be returning to coherence and also feeling and sensing as being framed in your attitude.

Now, since you have got some sense of the chakra which you aspire to stimulate and activate, let us understand the process to achieve the desired goal.

Breathing स्वाँस

Breathing exercise plays an important role in this chakra as holds true for all the other chakras. For achieving the desired stimulations in this chakra by breathing, sit in a relaxed manner in padma aasan पद्माआसन, and inhale and hold your breath in the lungs and feel the push (under no circumstances, you should try to hold it beyond your controllable limits). Subsequently, take that sense of push to your navel area and hold it there for as long as you can. Now, exhale very softly and slowly. Relax for a while before repeating the exercise again. Following the accomplishment of this exercise and anything less than having sweat on your forehead area, would not extend much benefits. So, would urge you to do it with full sincerity and for an extended period.

(Refer to Illustration 3.1: Padma Aasan पद्माआसन *at Page No. 68)*

Physical Yog योग
Uddiyan Bandh उद्यानबंध

For this aasan, you need to be standing straight with an erect back. Now, bend till the levels that your palms are resting on your bent knees. While maintaining this position, contract your belly inwards (do not engage breath to do this, it has to be contracted using the abdominal muscles only). It doesn't matter if you are not able to do it completely the first time. With regular practice, you would be able to perform it in the correct way. This aasan is believed to be extremely beneficial in improving digestion and curing constipation to a large extent.

(Refer to Illustration 3.2: Uddiyan Bandh उद्यानबंध *at Page No. 68)*

Kapalbhatti कपालभाटी

For performing this aasan, you can choose to be either in sidh aasan सिद्धआसन or padma aasan पद्माआसन. Increase the breathing rate, which means you have to inhale and exhale as fast you can. However, in both the cases, the muscles in your abdominal area should either contract or stretch. Doing this exercise without engagement of the abdominal muscle would be a waste of time and energy with no fruitful results. This exercise when done in a correct manner, helps in the release of toxins from body and also aids in relieving body and mind of stress.

(Refer to Illustration 3.3: **Kapalbhatti** कपालभाटी *at Page No. 69)*

Lom Vilom लोमविलोम

For this aasan also, you can choose to sit in either sidh aasan सिद्धआसन or padma aasan पद्माआसन. Engage your thumb to press your right nostril and inhale from the left nostril. Here onwards, while exhaling, use your ring and little finger to press the left nostril and breathe out from your right nostril. Repeat this exercise as many times as you can while maintaining the stretching and contraction stance of your abdominal muscles.

(Refer to Illustration 3.4: **Lom Vilom** लोमविलोम *at Page No. 69)*

Virbhadhra Aasan वीरभद्रआसन

This aasan derives its name from a form of Lord Shiva, namely, Virbhadhra. In this form, Lord Shiva is in an angry mood. For performing this aasan, stand straight with an erect back and then move your right leg forward and bend its knee. While holding this position, stretch your head with spread fingers of your hand over your head as if one is trying to catch something. Breathe fast and heavy while maintaining this pose. Continue the breathing as long as you can comfortably and then return to the standing position. Now, relax and repeat the exercise with left leg forward. Do ensure that the time period for both the legs remains the same and uniform number of breaths are inhaled and exhaled with either of leg stretched forward.

(Refer to Illustration 3.5: **Virbhadhra Aasan** वीरभद्रआसन *at Page No. 70)*

Viprit Virbhadhra Aasan विप्रीतवीरभद्रआसन

For performing this aasan, you need to be standing straight with an erect back. Now, from this position, stretch your legs sideways till you are comfortable holding on to that position. Now, turn your torso towards the right leg and raise your right hand above your head while keeping your left hand on the thigh or knee of the straight and stretched left leg and bend the right knee. Let your head follow your hand making and bend a little backwards as if you are watching the fingers of your right hand. Hold on to this position while maintaining a heavy and hard breathing. Hold as long as you are comfortable and then return to the position of stretched legs while keeping the torso straight. Relax before performing this exercise on the other side. This aasan has proven beneficial in providing strength to the legs, abdominal area and shoulders in addition to extending flexibility.

(Refer to Illustration 3.6: **Viprit Virbhadhra Aasan** विप्रीतवीरभद्रआसन *at Page No. 70)*

Trikon Aasan त्रिकोणआसन

For performing this aasan, you need to stand straight with an erect back. Now, stretch your legs sideways to the position as you are comfortable holding it there and able to balance yourself. While in this position, move your right arm to the back of your right leg in a manner that you are able to hold the heel of your right leg and move your left arm over your head and place your head in a position as if you are following your left arm and are able to see the fingers of your left hand. Hang on to this position while holding the breath inside you. Hold this position for as long as you can before returning to the standing position with your legs stretched sideways. Relax your body and try to breathe normally, before repeating this exercise on the other side. This aasan helps in improving digestion and provides great relief from stiff legs and hips and has also been found beneficial in easing sciatica pain.

(Refer to Illustration 3.7: **Trikon Aasan** त्रिकोणआसन *at Page No. 71)*

Ardh Chandra Aasan अर्धचंद्रआसन

For performing this aasan, you need to stand straight with an erect back. Following this, stretch your legs sideways. From this position, turn your torso towards the right side and bend the right knee, with your left leg almost stretched. Here onwards, bend your back forward and try to touch the ground on your right side with yourself facing the same way. Hold this position for as long as you can while ensuring that there is no breathlessness. Now return to the standing position with legs stretched sideways. Relax and repeat the exercise on the other side.

(Refer to Illustration 3.8: **Ardh Chandra Aasan** अर्धचंद्रआसन *at Page No. 71)*

Utihaprasarvkon Aasan उतिह्रापर्सर्वकोणआसन

For performing this aasan, you need to stand straight with an erect back and stretch your legs sideways in a comfortable position. Now, bend your right knee and with your right hand, the ground on the backside of the right foot and stretch your left hand over your head in such a manner as if you are trying to touch the ground (do not stretch too far as you may sustain injury; only stretch to the levels that you can hold for a good amount of time). Hold on to this position as long as you are comfortable with while maintaining normal breathing levels. Then, return to the standing position and relax and repeat the same exercise on the other side. This aasana gives strength to the shoulders, collar bone, and also improves chest strength.

(Refer to Illustration 3.9: **Utihaprasarvkon Aasan** उतिह्रापर्सर्वकोणआसन *at Page No. 72)*

Phalaasan पलआसन

For performing this aasan, lie down on your belly and lift yourself with bended elbows in an effort to form a plank. Try and keep your entire body in a straight line and keep your head in a forward looking position while keeping your breath normal. Maintain this position as per your comfort levels without feeling breathlessness. This aasana increases the strength of abdominal muscles in addition to strengthening legs, chest and shoulders.

(Refer to Illustration 3.10: **Phalaasan** पलआसन *at Page No. 72)*

Vashishth Aasan वशिष्ठआसन

For performing this aasan, you need to lie on your high side. Now, lift your body sideways using the right hand. Lift your body till the time the right hand becomes fully stretched and keep your feet joined, with one placed over the other.

(Refer to Illustration 3.11: **Vashishth Aasan** वशिष्ठआसन *at Page No. 73)*

Salbhas Aasan सलभसआसन

For performing this aasan, you need to lie down on your belly with arms around the waist area. From this position, lift your head, chest and legs while keeping your arms in the air. Hold on to this position for a while and try sustaining your breath as long as you can comfortably. Now, return to the first position of lying down on your belly. Relax for a while before repeating the exercise.

(Refer to Illustration 3.12: **Salbhas Aasan** सलभसआसन *at Page No. 73)*

Hand Formulations बंध

As described earlier, this chakra has "fire" as the most dominating element. Among the fingers, the element of fire is represented by the ring finger. However, as is universal, the same holds true for bandha बंध too. For any energy to have any form, it needs to have at least earth, which in the case of fingers is the "thumb". Accordingly, we form the surya mudra by touching tips of the ring finger and that of the thumb while keeping the breathing heavy, which means inhale more and exhale slowly. There is no holding of the breath involved in this.

(Refer to Illustration 3.13: **Hand Formulations** बंध *[Surya Mudra] at Page No. 74)*

Focus-based Exercises ध्यानक्रिया

For dhayan yog ध्यानयोग़, you need to sit in a comfortable position either in an aasan or in a chair or something else. Take deep breaths and exhale slowly and then gently start holding onto your breath and try and push the breath to your belly (navel area) and hold it there. You should/may feel some tingling sensations around your navel. Now, slowly release the breath. The time when you are holding your breath in the belly area, try and keep your unhindered focus there only.

Mantra Recitation मंत्रउच्चारण

There are ten major phonemes in this chakra.

RRNRNRNRNRARARARARRMRMRMRMMMM

Reciting in the above manner seems to have yielded better results as in regards to unblocking and stimulating of the manipura chakra. Prefer doing this recitation while sitting on the floor (you may use some kind of cushion for sitting) on an empty stomach. This is necessary for the simple reason that when recitation is executed, it should always be done on an empty stomach, as that is the time when the enzymes are at the optimum level and secondly the body is hydrated and water element is not being exercised for digesting food.

Naad Kriya ध्रुनीयोग

To be able to perform this ध्रुनीयोग, you need to be in the most comfortable position—physically, biologically, and psychologically. Try and focus in and around your navel area, not from outside but from within the skeleton. Subsequently, try and get your hearing senses to the area of navel where the movement of energies could be heard. Keep yourself glued to that movement and hear it for as long you can.

Yantra Sadhna यंत्रसाधना

As described in the first chapter on chakra, you may choose to form the yantra of kundalini by using your own body, which is the common yantra for all the chakras. This is so because this yantra helps in creating and clearing the path for the kundalini to move above from the tail of the spine to the uppermost part of the skull.

Illustrative Representation of Aasana's

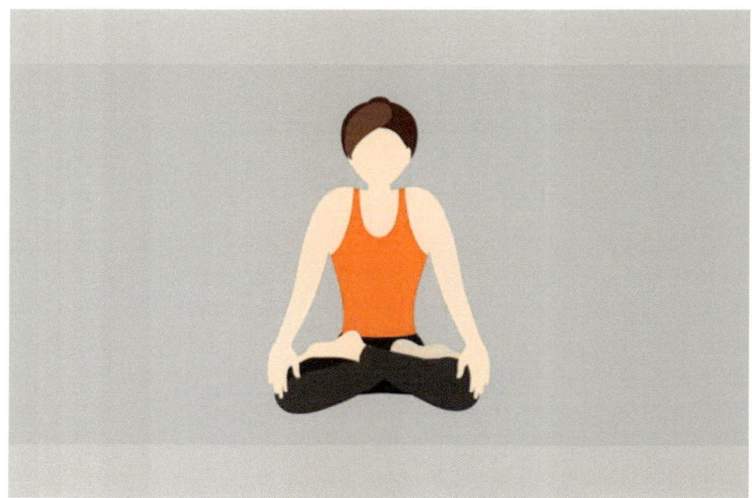

Illustration 3.1: Sidh Aasan सिद्धआसन

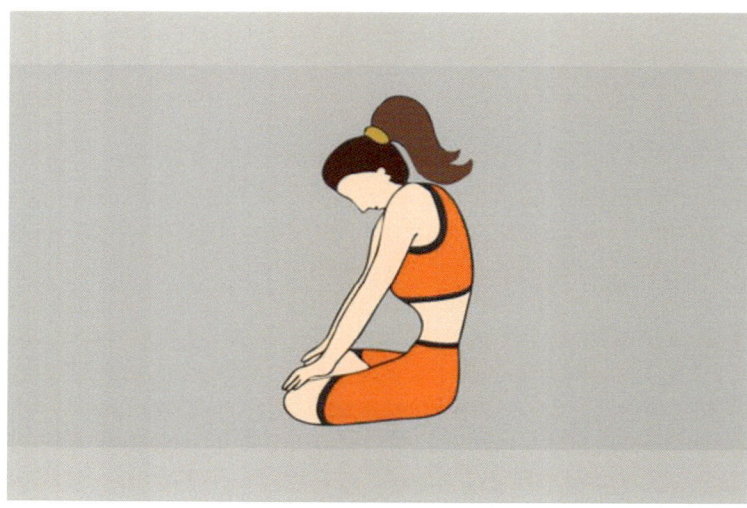

Illustration 3.2: Uddiyan Bandh उड्यानबंध

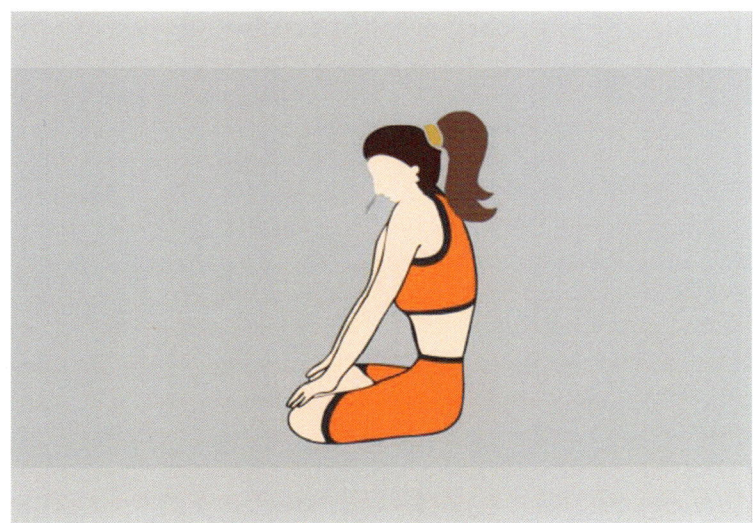

Illustration 3.3: Kapalbhatti कपालभाटी

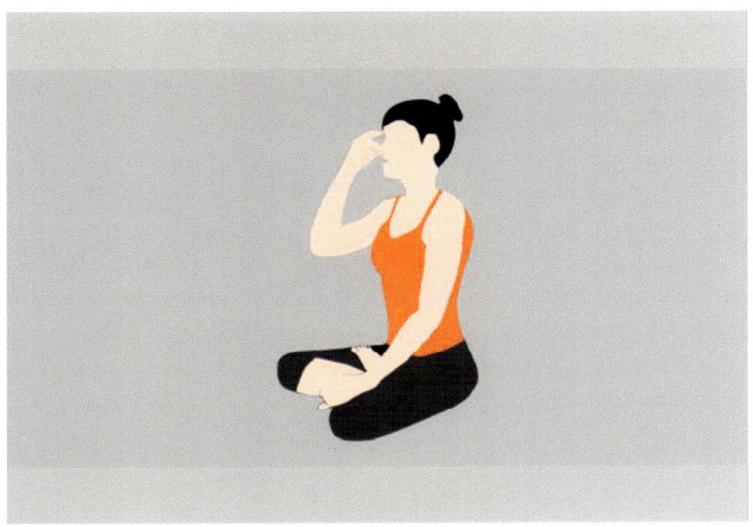

Illustration 3.4: Lom Vilom लोमविलोम

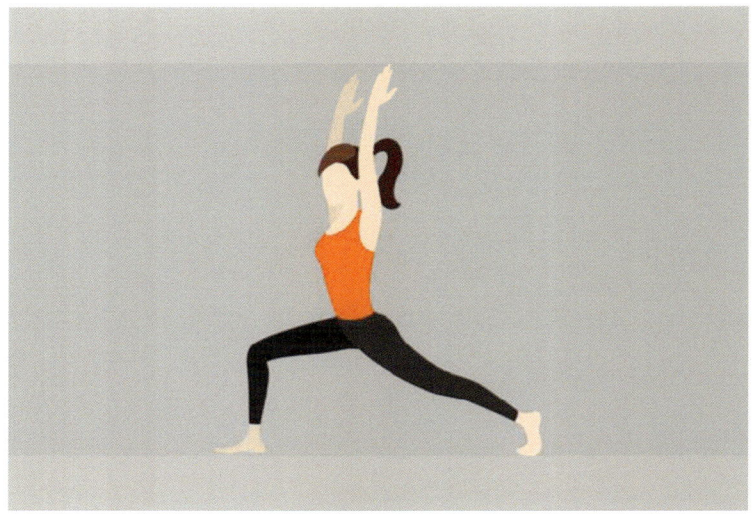

Illustration 3.5: Virbhadhra Aasan वीरभद्रआसन

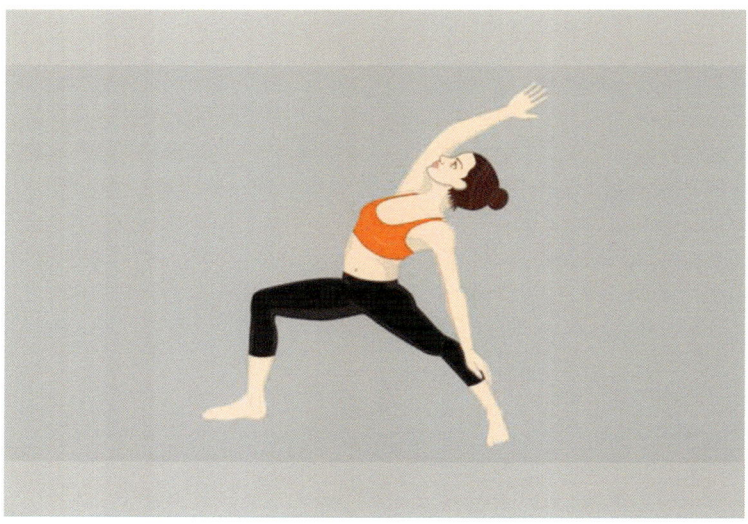

Illustration 3.6: Viprit Virbhadhra Aasan विप्रीतवीरभद्रआसन

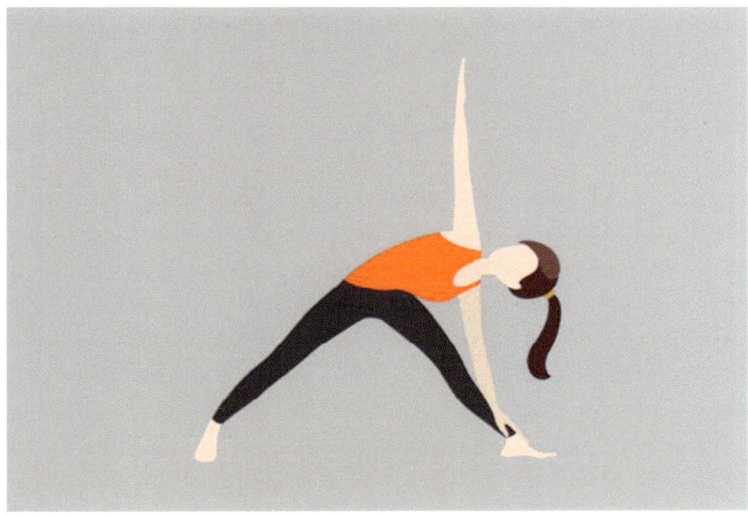

Illustration 3.7: Trikon Aasan त्रिकोणआसन

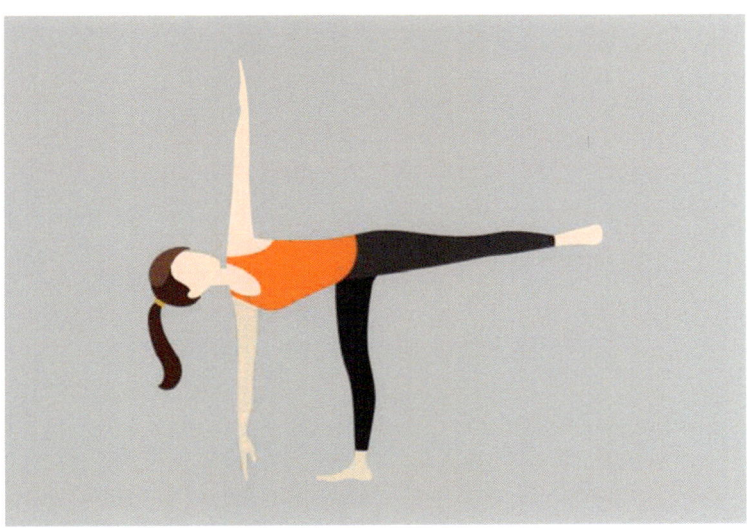

Illustration 3.8: Ardh Chandra Aasan अर्धचंद्रआसन

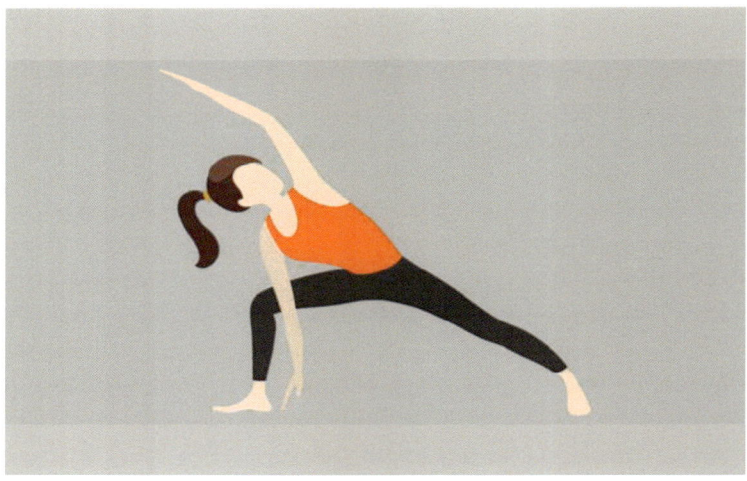

Illustration 3.9: Utihaprasarvkon Aasan उतिहापर्सर्वकोणआसन

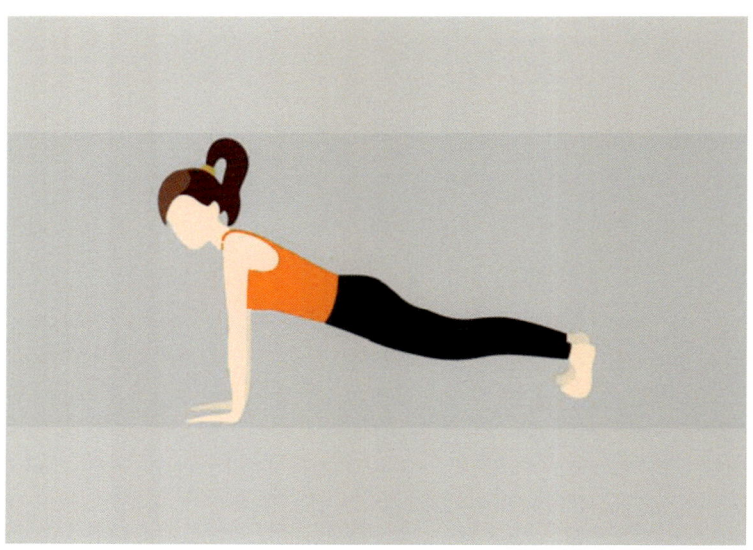

Illustration 3.10: Phalaasan पलआसन

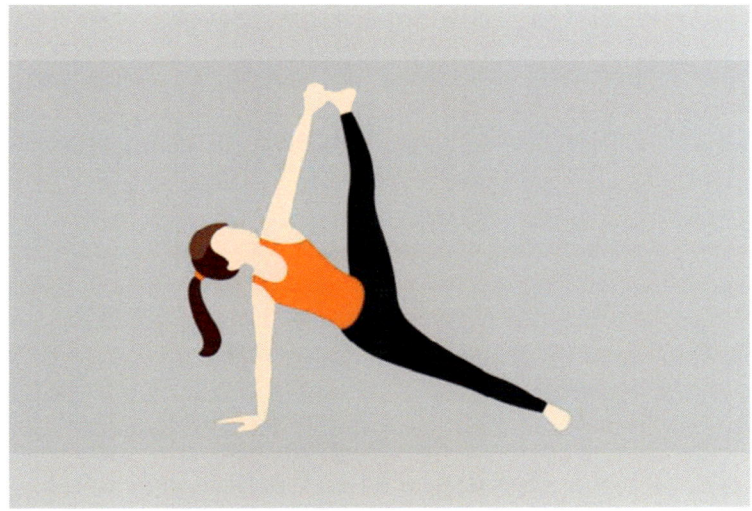

Illustration 3.11: Vashishth Aasan वशिष्ठआसन

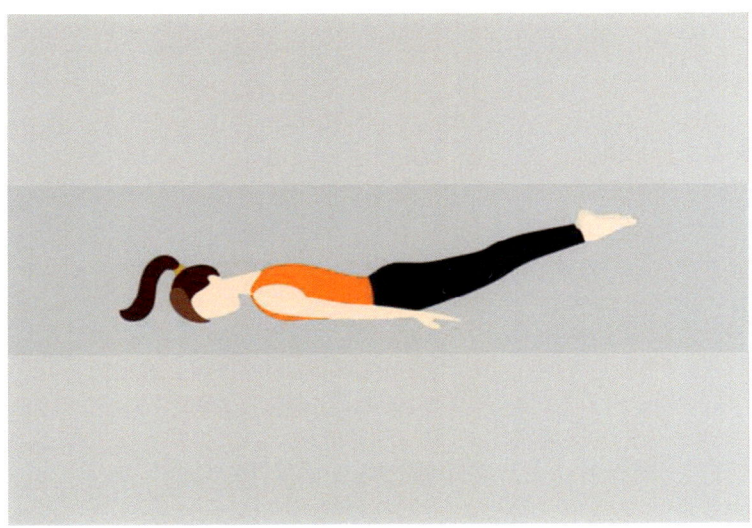

Illustration 3.12: Salbhas Aasan सलभसआसन

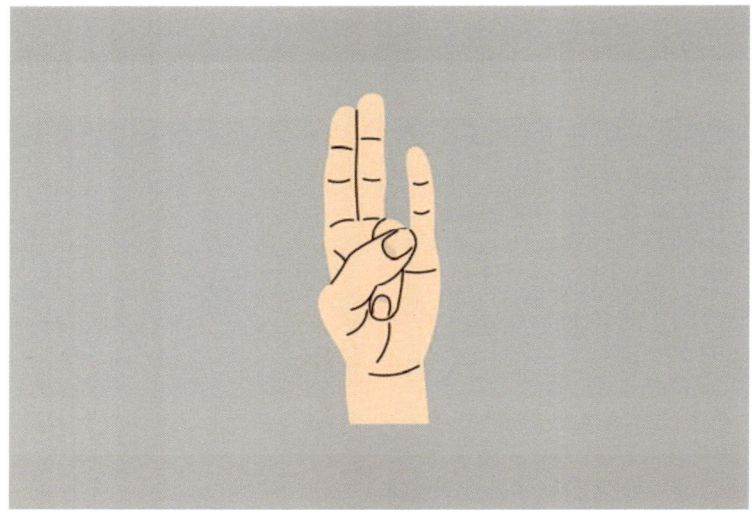

Illustration 3.13: Hand Formulations बंध [Surya Mudra]

4

Swadisthana Chakra: Controlling the Water Element of the Body

As the title suggests, this chakra defines, assimilates and controls water element of the body. The percentage share of water element in the body is approximately 75, as is the case with mother earth. Element water is the most prudent and influential one, defining emotions, their reactions and also how and what would be the possibilities of your movements in the society, family and other facets of life. This chakra should not be understood as a place where this element is hosted or as a kind of reservoir, but instead, this chakra has the confluence points which define/regulate this element. Additionally, this element has the ability to respond to other poignant energies, which may be embodied or disembodied or visible or invisible—as what influences you, may not necessarily be visible to the eye. For example, the air which defines the temperature is not visible. Likewise, there are so many energies which are not visible to the naked eye but are still poignant). The Sanskrit name for this chakra is swadisthana chakra स्वाधिष्ठानचक्र where your being is established. "Swa" means self and "disthana" means established.

मेरुबह्याप्रदेसेससीमिहिरसिरेसव्यदकसेनिसन्नेमध्येनाडीसुसुमनातृतीया-
गुनामयीकंदरायाचिराशटाधतूरा-समेरा-पुस्पाग्रथीता-
तमावापुहकंदमध्याचिराशटावज्ञाख्यामेधरदेस:चिराशिपरिगत: मध्यमेस:
ज्वलनती:

The aforementioned verse in Sanskrit, for the sake of understanding the ethos of what is being said and referred, would broadly translate to:

In the space outside the Meru, placed on the left and the right, are the two Siras, Sasi and Mihira. The nadi sushmna, whose substance is the threefold Gunas, is in the middle. She is a form of moon, sun, and fire. Her body, a string of blooming Dhatura flowers, extends to the middle of the Kanda to the head, and the Vajra inside her extends, shining from the Medhra to the head.

The techniques enshrined in the Vedas are targeted towards not only strengthening one particular element but rather how to balance all the elements in the body to have presumptuous gains. That being the ethos, the metal associated with this chakra is gold, which is hot in nature and is said to stimulate heat/fire within the body. Wearing gold when the water element is imbalanced depends on what is desired by an individual; in the sense of aspirations an individual would like to pursue in life. However, if one is aspiring to excel in the spiritual world, then inexorably, gold is not the metal that one should be wearing. However, if one is having issues with the growth path in career, wearing of gold would be conducive.

Talking further about the confluence points, this chakra is host to two types of energies, namely, the energy coming from the root chakra which is kind of already established and defined and the other energies coalescent with this point emanating from other parts of the body. As a result, this chakra is perceived more prudent as the energy released by this chakra post assimilation, would be having its effect on the other chakras as well in addition to affecting the root chakra. Significantly, this defines as to what would be the nature of further transmissions from the root chakra.

The pronouncements from this chakra define the taste worthiness on your tongue. Simply putting, if you feel tasteless, recourse to unblocking the sacral chakra would be the best way to overcome it. Mostly, this tasteless virtue develops, post-intensive medication and of lately, as to what is being observed in the case of people getting inflicted with Covid-19. Since the taste generally, and of life, is governed by this chakra, one can assume that the intimate relationships and desires are also governed by this chakra. So, if you are feeling hapless about the fervour in life, you need to approach this chakra and cure it to have the sense of rejoicing.

This chakra controls and regulates apaan vayu आपानवायू which is responsible for the excretory functions (like sweat, urine etc.) and in ladies, it has an additional role in creating a safe passage for the foetus during the delivery. Prithvi mudra is a mudra for this chakra, which is formed by joining the tips of the thumb and the ring finger. This chakra, as mentioned above, controls the emotions apart from associating with the warmth in that emotion. Intensity of love and prejudice is also defined by this chakra.

This chakra has six inlets/outlets, creating 6 major and 38 minor notes of sound during the receiving, assimilation and transfer of energy, and is mild red in colour. The six petals represent the following modes of consciousness, also known as *vrittis*: affection, pitilessness, feeling of all-destructiveness, delusion, disdain, and suspicion.

Swadisthana is often associated with pleasure, sense of oneself, relationships, sensuality and procreation. Its element is water and the colour is orange. It is blocked by guilt. Swadisthana is associated with the unconscious and emotions. It is closely related to the mooldhara. Mooldhara is where the different *samskaras* (potential karmas) lie dormant, and swadisthana is where these samskaras find expression.

Swadisthana encompasses the unconscious desires, especially the sexual desire. It is often conveyed that raising the kundalini shakti (energy of consciousness) above Swadisthana is difficult. Many Hindu saints have had to face sexual temptations associated with this chakra.

One who meditates on swadisthana is believed to have acquired the following *siddhis,* viz. freedom from enemies, the status of a lord among the yogis, eloquence and clarity (the flow of words resonating like nectar in a well-reasoned discourse), awareness of astral entities and the ability to taste anything desired for oneself or others. Lord Vishnu is the presiding devta देवता, since he is worshipped as the god who takes care of life and the life belongings and this chakra, plays a similar role in life. The beej mantras associated with Lord Vishnu are the ones which are recited for the stimulation and activation of this chakra which makes a person punctual and adhering to the timings. Coming late and not sticking to the time schedules is also an indication of dysfunctional sacral chakra.

In addition to the taste and fervour, this chakra is also significantly responsible for the sensory aspects of the body. The way one perceives and conceives a situation and the corresponding reaction to those situations is more or less defined and governed by this sacral chakra. We can comfortably deduce that a defined behaviour and action pertaining to this chakra is quite crucial for a successful and impactful societal life. In addition, if one desires to make it large in life, especially in the field of creativity, or for that matter, even to have the ability to express oneself, one shouldn't be ignoring this chakra at all. It won't be wrong to mention or conclude that this chakra encompasses the possibilities to either make or break. If functional at an optimum level, the person would have all the desired virtues of life, would be appreciated and would garner accolades. However, if this chakra exhibits dysfunctionality, it can result in irritation and negative thinking in a person— schadenfreude/epicaricacy being the dominant emotion.

Pertinently, this chakra is helpful in designing and drawing a framework of life that one desires. Therefore, it is important that this ever-important foundational chakra is not neglected. Many illnesses that can originate from this energy center are manifest simply due to the fear of losing control of our relationships with others and even our binding to physical engagements like business deals or projects we are closely attached to.

A person's desires, needs, longings, and urges arise from this chakra. In other words, this chakra facilitates what you experience through your senses—pleasurable or uncomfortable—things that you want and the things for which you aren't appreciative about. The chakras function as a sort of limbic system, although working in tandem, yet their motions may not be corresponding to the next in order, but rather can be opposite in direction. This limbic system processes all the experiences and consequently results in secretion of joy or sorrow. This chakra contributes emotions to the limbic system. In psychological terms, sacral chakra guides a person towards sense of satisfaction. Spiritually, it instigates the urge of connecting with the energies in higher dimensions, in addition to providing a sense of solace and harmony within, thereby resulting in emotional stability. The ability to sense deeper and hidden emotions is the key to realisation and activation of sacral chakra. As it is, these unexpressed emotions are kind of responsible for it to be blocked in the first place (these emotions could be owed to your own understanding about the situations in life or the cynical remarks aired by others).

Challenges arise when we experience the inability to create physical expressions of our life outside the familial authority of the first chakra. In such a scenario, we are bringing baggage from the mooldhara into our sacral chakra. Imbalances in sacral chakra can manifest in low confidence, lack of motivation, inability to create intimate connection with others, lack of interest in self-expression or artistic abilities, infertility, urinary problems, difficulties in giving birth, producing orgasms and low libido.

Prevalence of a certain tendency has been observed regards the stretching of system beyond its existing limits, guided by the emotion of "no pain no gain". This principle may be true and relevant otherwise but not in yog. A blend of sense and sensations is necessary and one should always avoid any sort of pain whilst undertaking any of the yog postures. May it be physical or related to breathing there should never be a sentiment of stretching beyond one's comfortable limits. The sensation of awareness and consciousness should always prevail. However, if there is a pain in the body, the awareness has been compromised and hence the results so attained from the exercises too have been compromised.

A few of the common health problems which are fallout of an imbalanced sacral chakra include:
- Chronic lower back pain
- Arthritis
- Genital or sexual problems
- Hip issues

Swadisthana is located at two finger-widths above the mooldhara chakra मूलाधार or the root chakra which is located in the coccyx (tailbone). Its corresponding *kshetram* or "place" is in the front of the body, barely below the belly button. It is connected with the sense of taste (the tongue) and reproduction (the genitals). It is often associated with the testes and the ovaries. They produce hormones viz. testosterone or estrogen, which influence the sexual behaviour. They are stored in areas where genetic information lies dormant, much like the way the samskaras समस्कार lie dormant within the swadisthana.

The endeavour of undertaking the exercises should first be understood before putting them into practice. The ethos of all the exercises/yog for this chakra is to align the grounded energy (mooldhara) with sushumna nadi सुषुम्नानाड़ी, which is the only polarity you have to connect body with the cosmic.

Post realising and knowing as to what you are about to engage into, let me tell you the processes by which you would be able stimulate the sacral chakra. As mentioned in the previous chapter, there are several paths that you may choose, to achieve your goal of activating the sacral chakra. These are:
1. Breathing स्वाँस

2. Physical Yog योग
3. Hand Formulations बंध
4. Focus-based Exercises ध्यानक्रिया
5. Mantras Recitation मंत्रउच्चारण
6. Naad Kriya ध्वनीयोग
7. Yantra Sadhna यंत्रसाधना
8. Tantra Sadhna तंत्रसाधना

Now, I shall walk you along all of these processes for stimulating and hence activating the sacral chakra.

Breathing स्वाँस

Breath, which is the essence of living, is equally prudent in its attribute so far as kundalini yog is concerned and holds true even for the sacral chakra. For the stimulation of this chakra, following are the steps which you must adopt:

(a) Sense the inhaling of your breath.
(b) Follow your breath till the lungs (do not forget to observe the back of lungs too).
(c) Feel the change and effects, transpiring because of the breath.
(d) Follow the breath back to your nostrils till the time it is thrown out of the system.

You need to be observant at all times as any wavering during the process would deprive you of the developments. Importantly, at any point of time, you should not try altering the normal pace of breathing.

Physical Yog योग

Before you embark upon the physical exercises, yog, kindly adhere to the following so that you are in harmony with yourself and the results obtained post the exercises should extend a comforting feeling instead of causing anxiety.

1. Place yourself in sidh aasan सिद्धआसन (you may start by sitting with a rigid back so that the spine is erect, and both your feet are touching the ground).
2. Now with your pelvis, try and push yourself downwards and simultaneously, with your shoulders and chest, try to lift yourself (don't get up, just exert the force).
3. While maintaining the position as mentioned in point 2, try and hold your breath and while releasing it, exhale it from your mouth, enacting it as a "vomiting" action. Now, repeat the breathing process at least five times in the above described manner to ease yourself from any thoughts or stress in order to comprehend with yourself and motions in the body.

(Refer to Illustration 4.1: **Sidh Aasan** सिद्धआसन *at Page No. 90)*

Supt Badhakon Aasan सुसबधकोणआसन

This aasan is helpful in improving the productive health, both in men and women, in addition to providing relief from stiff hip as it helps in lubricating the pelvis and the hip area.

This aasana can be performed by the starters by following the below two steps:
1) Lie down comfortably on your back with a stretched out position to the front.
2) Now bend your knees while lying on your back in such a manner so as to form the shape of a flower vas. Further, stretch your arms out with palms facing upwards but keeping them below the shoulder level.

Now, try to touch the knees of the bent legs with each other while maintaining the bent position. Try to inhale when touching the knees together and exhale while bringing back the legs on to the ground. At no point, you should experience any sort of stress, may it be during the stretching or while contracting and touching of the knees or while breathing. The objective is to remain calm and relaxed during the entire course of exercise and avoid stress. It is not necessary or mandatory that you should be able to complete the entire exercise from the very onset. Slowly, as you gain strength and energy, you would be able to complete the exercise by its very own ethics.

(Refer to Illustration 4.2: **Supt Badhakon Aasan** सुप्तबद्धकोणआसन *at Page No. 90)*

Anand Baal Aasan आनंदबालआसन

This aasana is more or less inspired from a child, who rejoices the sense of being alive and while enjoying this jubilation, tends to feel the physical organs by touching them. This aasan is beneficial in lessening pain during the menstruation cycle, especially in the teen age and is also helpful in augmenting hunger. In this aasan, the stretching and contraction is targeted towards touching the heels of the feet with palms when the arms are stretched out. There is no alteration of breath and no feel of sagacity in the physical body.

For performing this aasan, lie on your back and bend your knees, with your legs raised from the ground. Now grope your legs with your arms from the inner side of the legs and try and hold/touch the heels of your feet. Hold onto this position while breathing normally. Hereafter, try and pull your legs towards your shoulders while maintaining a "no stress" sentiment and any heaviness in your breath. Maintain this position for a while before releasing your legs and lying down on your back in a relaxed position. Repeat this exercise for at least five to seven times before moving onto the next one.

During the course, initially you may experience some rigidity in legs and thighs but it should not be a matter of concern as one would be able to overcome it with regular practice schedules. However, I do repeat, under no circumstances, you should stretch yourself to the levels whereby pain or stress is felt. Supposedly, that would prove detrimental in familiarizing yourself with the awareness of the body and the sense of enjoyment of the aasana.

(Refer to Illustration 4.3: **Anand Baal Aasan** आनंदबालआसन *at Page No. 91)*

Jathraparivart Aasan ज्ठरापरिवर्तआसन

In this aasan, lie down on your back with arms stretched out at shoulder height. Now while lying, bend your knee and pull up the leg towards your chest. While the leg is airborne, try to place yourself on the ground on the opposite side with the bent knee. While maintaining this position, tilt your head in the opposite side from the side of the bent knee. Hold your body in this stretched position while ensuring that the comfort level is not compromised with any related stress. Repeat this exercise for the other leg too whilst ascertaining all the other prescribed details, including the head to tilt in the opposite direction from the bent knee.

This aasana is advantageous in relieving strain and stress in the spine and pelvis area, and is also helpful in improving digestion and hunger enhancement.

(Refer to Illustration 4.4: **Jathraparivart Aasan** ज्ठरापरिवर्तआसन *at Page No. 91)*

Badhakon Aasan बधकोणआसन

This aasan is performed while maintaining a sitting posture. Sit on the floor with an erect back and bend your knees by joining your feet together. While placed in this position, compress your knees further with your feet joined to each other towards the groin area (the extent of the compression should be comfortable and at no instance should you injure your inner thighs). Hold onto this position till the time you don't get breathless or feel heaviness while breathing. Maintain the posture before returning to the position of front legs fully stretched. Relax for a while before repeating the exercise. For the starters, it would be advisable to monitor their stretching ability. Feel the contentment of your stretching limits till the time you are able to bring your feet near the groin area and your knees are able to touch the ground.

This aasana is beneficial in rectifying discomforts in the hips and pelvis area while stimulating the groin area. Improvement in digestion is another added benefit.

(Refer to Illustration 4.5: **Badhakon Aasan** बधकोणआसन *at Page No. 92)*

Upavistha Konaasan उपविष्टाकोणआसन

In this aasan, you have to stretch your legs sideways while being placed in a sitting position. Hereafter, bend forward to touch the ground with your chest. While touching the ground with your chest, try and grip the thumb of your feet. Hold onto this position for a while without any undue stress in the back, pelvis, groin and inner thigh areas. Now, release the grip and return to your sitting posture with legs stretched sideways. Relax for a while before repeating the exercise. Additionally, do exercise caution not to stress yourself; for completing the posture at the very onset, would involve rigorous training before it can be achieved.

This aasana helps in removing blockages in the groin area while providing flexibility to the hips. It would also strengthen your back to facilitate a correct posture.

(Refer to Illustration 4.6: **Upavistha Konaasan** उपविष्टाकोणआसन *at Page No. 92)*

Agnisthamb Aasan अग्निस्तम्भआसन

In this aasan, you need to sit down on the floor with an erect back. Hereafter, place your left shin over your right thigh. There could be issues with people having stiff back or hips. However, over a period of time, they would be able to inculcate the flexibility to perform this aasana. When you have managed to put your shin on the thigh, try reaching out to the floor with hands and touch the same. Now, aiming at touching the ground with your chest, use your hands to repulse this movement. To mention again, do not strain yourself beyond the comfortable limits. Maintain this posture as long as there is no stress in the body and no heaviness in the breath is evident. At an advanced level, you can attempt to hold onto your breath by inhaling more and holding the breath for a longer period of time. While sustaining this posture, try to hold yourself without any breath, meaning no inhaling for a brief period of time after exhaling.

This aasan has been assumed helpful in easing stiffness in the hips and the pelvis area in addition to providing stimulation to the naadi नाड़ी, which is instrumental in facilitating energy towards the sacral chakra from the root chakra. This aasan shall also provide strength to your back to enable long duration meditation.

(Refer to Illustration 4.7: **Agnisthamb Aasan** अग्निस्तम्भआसन *at Page No. 93)*

Uttan Aasan उत्तासआसन

This aasan would hold its validity for the first four chakras, as mentioned and illustrated in the previous chapter on root chakra. For this chakra, there is a variation in the way one is supposed to perform this aasan. The holding period and stretching would be more in comparison to what you would undergo in the case of muldhara chakra.

(Refer to Illustration 4.8: **Uttan Aasan** उत्तासआसन *at Page No. 93)*

Adho Mukha Aasan आधमुख्बासआसन

As is the case with uttan aasan उत्तासआसन, even this aasan would be repeated for stimulation and activation of this chakra, with a variation in the placement of legs. For this chakra, the legs have to be spread wider in comparison to their stance in the root chakra. Moreover, you are expected to hold your breath during the entire period of this posture with the remaining procedures continuing to be the same.

(Refer to Illustration 4.9: **Adho Mukha Aasan** आधमुख्बासआसन *at Page No. 94)*

Anjaney Aasan आंजनेयआसन

In this aasan, the stretching of the back would be done with assistance from chest, shoulders and arms. While standing in an erect position, move your right leg forward and bend it while keeping the left leg stretched in the same position. With a bent right leg and a stretched left leg, try to stretch your straight arms towards the back and hold your breath while maintaining the position. At no point, you should outstretch yourself beyond the comfortable limits or feel breathless. Now, release the position and return to the standing one. Relax for a while and repeat the exercise by interchanging the posture of legs—left leg would now be in the bent position and the right leg would be in the stretched position. The backward movement and stretching of the arms would remain the same as would be holding of the breath for that period.

This aasana is beneficial in clearing the nerve blockings, in addition to easing stiffness in the shoulders, and providing relief and strength to the cervical.

(Refer to Illustration 4.10: **Anjaney Aasan** आंजनेयआसन *at Page No. 94)*

Uttanpristh Aasan उत्तानपृष्ठआसन

For performing this aasan, lie down on your chest with legs fully stretched out. Now, pull back your arms and bend your elbows, with legs in a stretched position. While resting the upper torso on your bent elbows and legs being stretched out, bend your right leg and try bringing it close to your chest. Hold onto this position while maintaining breathing at a normal pace. You can now return back to the resting position with your chest touching the ground. Repeat the above process by engaging the other leg, trying to touch the chest.

(Refer to Illustration 4.11: **Uttanpristh Aasan** उत्तानपृष्ठआसन *at Page No. 95)*

Ekpaskot Aasan एकपसकोत

In this aasan, lie down on your back with arms comfortably resting by the side of your body. Now, bend both your legs and touch base of both the feet, forming a kind of triangle. Hold this position for a while before releasing it. Repeat the exercise for almost ten to twelve times. This aasan is rewarding in controlling and regulating water element in the body. This aasan may also be chosen in case of hyper anxiety following due consultation with the doctor.

(Refer to Illustration 4.12: **Ekpaskot Aasan** एकपसकोत *at Page No. 95)*

Hand Formulations

Surya mudra सूर्यमुद्रा is formed by joining the tips of thumb and the ring finger. This can be performed while sitting in sidh aasan सिद्धआसन or in padmaaasan पद्माआसन. Inhale almost double the air than your normal capacity and hold the breath in your belly by protruding it outwards.

Maintain this position as long as you can and then gently exhale, taking thrice the time of what was employed while inhaling. *Would strongly recommend seeking medical opinion about your physical health, before initiating this exercise.*

(Refer to Illustration 4.13: **Hand Formulations** [Surya Mudra] *at Page No. 96*)

Mantra Recitation

The mantra for this chakra is to be recited while exhaling

VNVNVNVNVNVNVNANANANANANVANVANVANVAMVA
MVAM

The duration as to how you can recite the mantra at one go, would entirely depend upon the strength of this chakra. You can start by reciting small notes of this mantra and continue as per your comfort level.

Naad Kriya नादयोग़

In this, the focus has to be drawn towards the swadisthana chakra and subsequently, the confluence is observed and recognized by hearing to the phonemes created by the handshake and handoffs. To recognise the same, the chakra has to be activated and should be in full strength.

Anything deficient won't bring in the desired results—either you won't be able to hear anything at all and even if you do hear by forcing yourself onto it, it would be nothing more than a "hallucination".

Swadisthana Chakra: Controlling the Water Element of...

Yantra Sadhna यंत्रसाधना

The physical body yantra for this chakra and in fact for all the chakras is the same. You may prefer doing the physical exercise of forming the yantra, and then implement any of the prescribed ways to activate your swadisthana chakra.

Tantra Sadhna तंत्रसाधना

As mentioned in the previous chapter, while administering this procedure, it would be better to have the physical presence and guidance of a teacher. I would abstain in highlighting any of the tantric procedures out here because these procedures don't leave you with the levy of error, and anything performed inaccurately would be detrimental in nature. Kindly seek the advice of your teacher/guru, and attempt to do this step in their presence.

Illustrative Representation of Aasana's

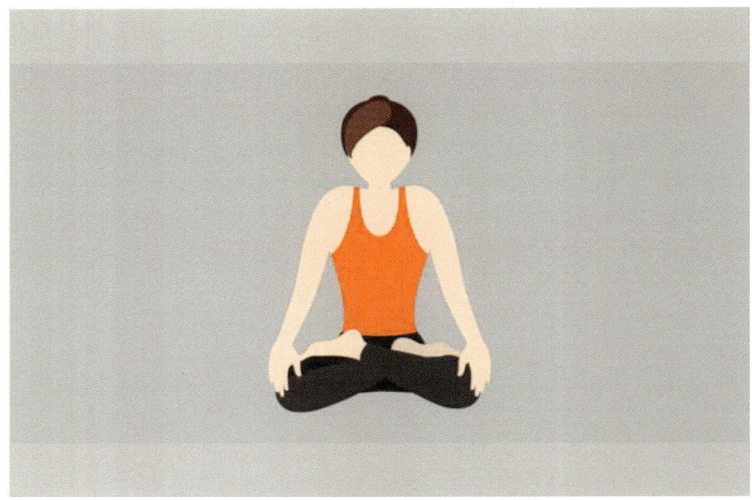

Illustration 4.1: Sidh Aasan सिद्धआसन

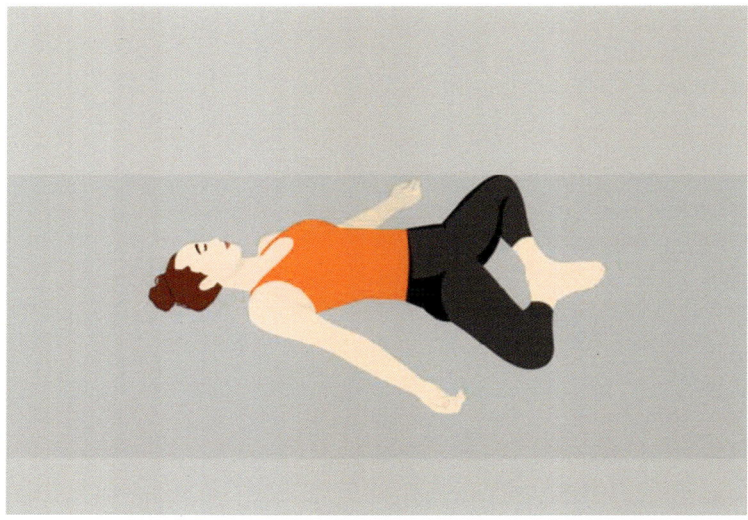

Illustration 4.2: Supt Badhakon Aasan सुप्तबधकोणआसन

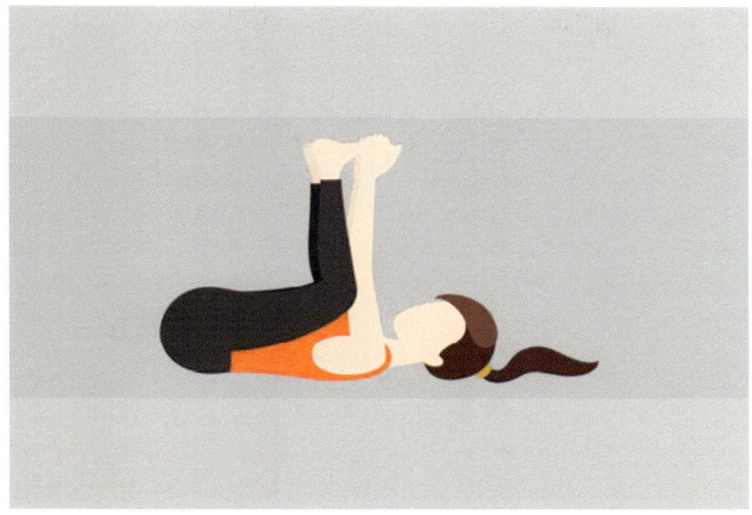

Illustration 4.3: Anand Baal Aasan आनंदबालआसन

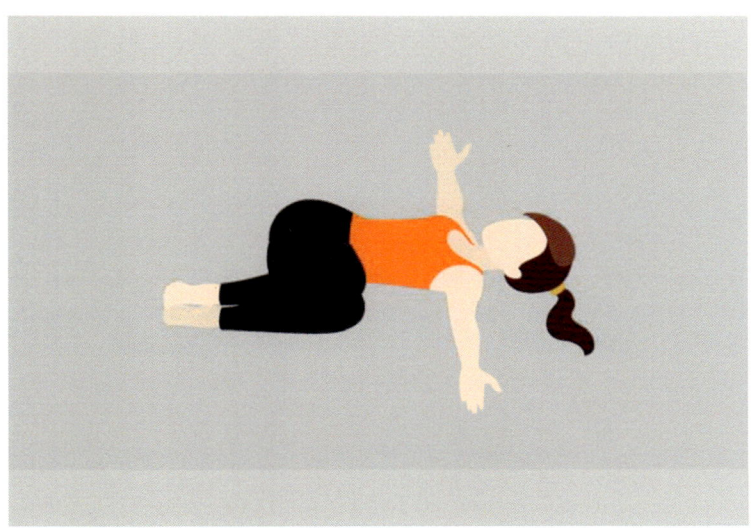

Illustration 4.4: Jathraparivart Aasan ज्ठरापरिवर्तआसन

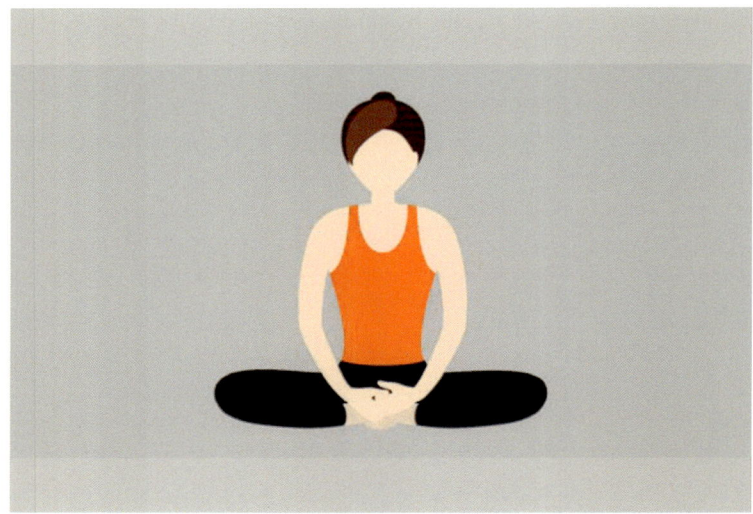

Illustration 4.5: Badhakon Aasan बध्दकोणआसन

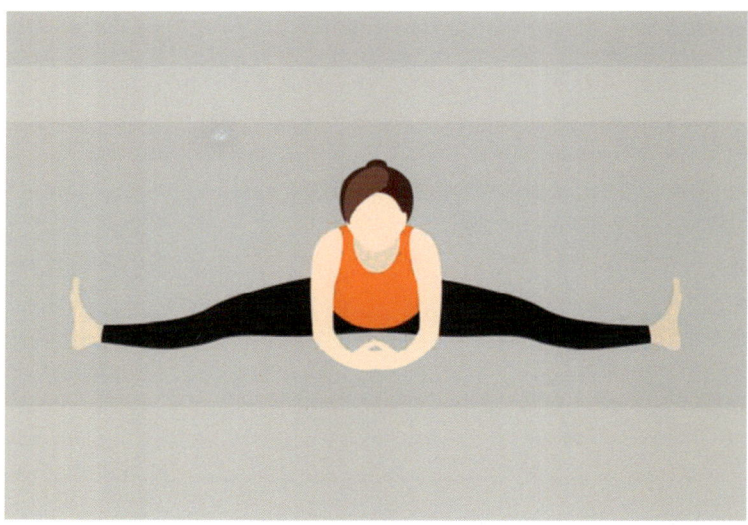

Illustration 4.6: Upavistha Konaasan उपविष्ठाकोणआसन

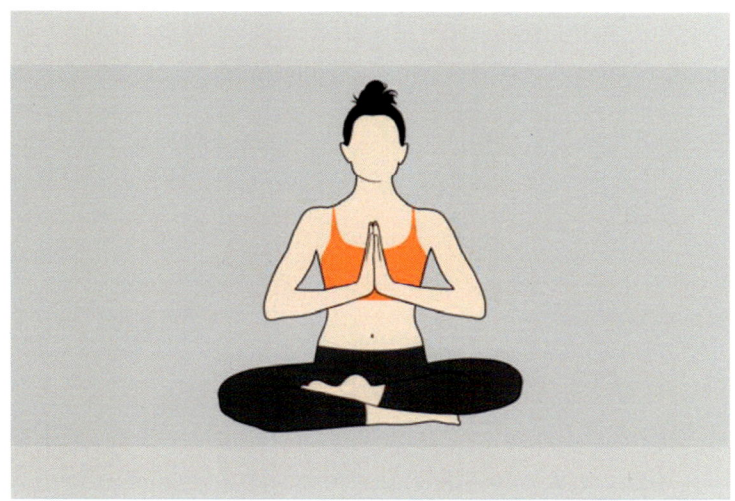

Illustration 4.7: Agnisthamb Aasan अग्निस्तम्भआसन

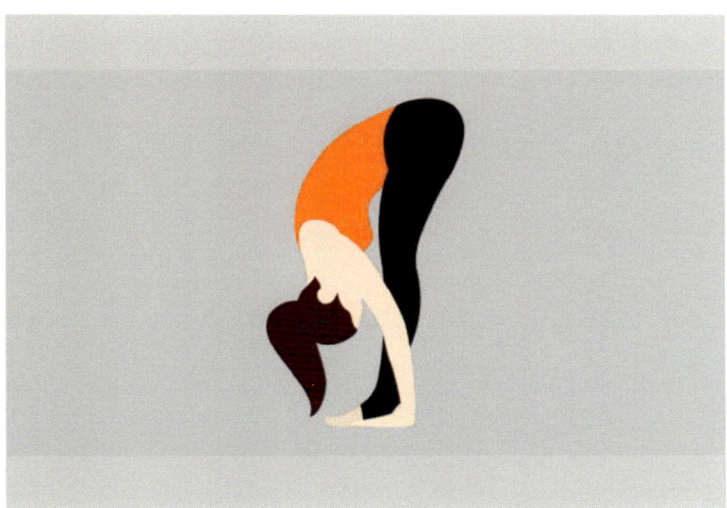

Illustration 4.8: Uttan Aasan उत्तासआसन

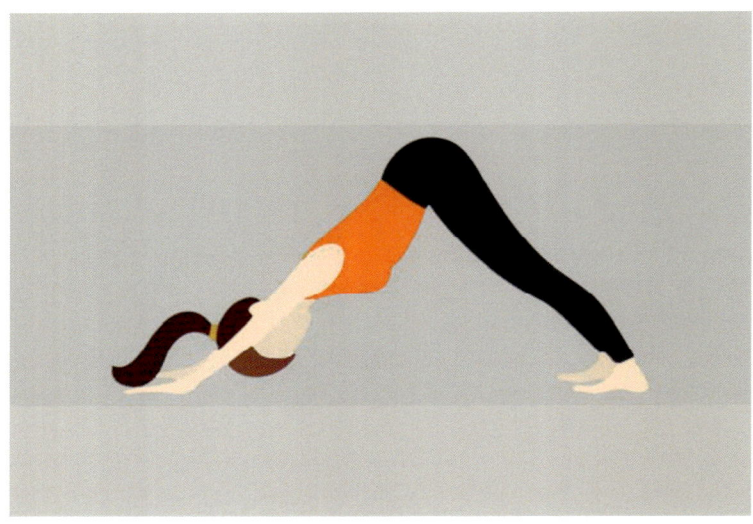

Illustration 4.9: Adho Mukha Aasan आध्मुख्वासआसन

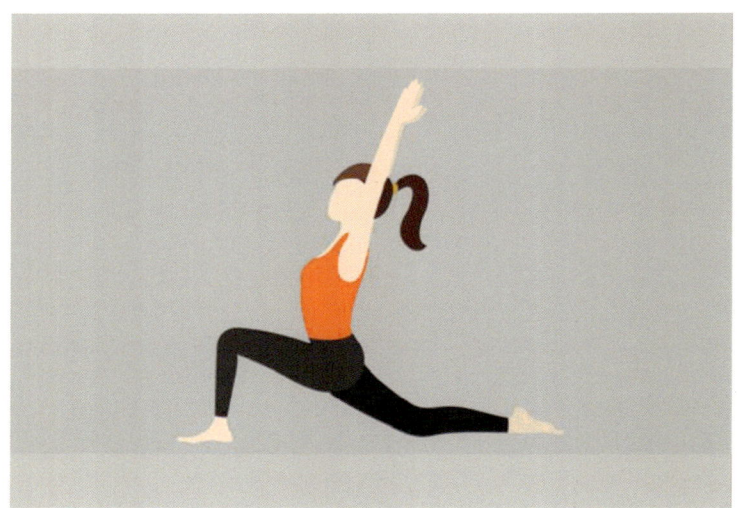

Illustration 4.10: Anjaney Aasan आंजनेयआसन

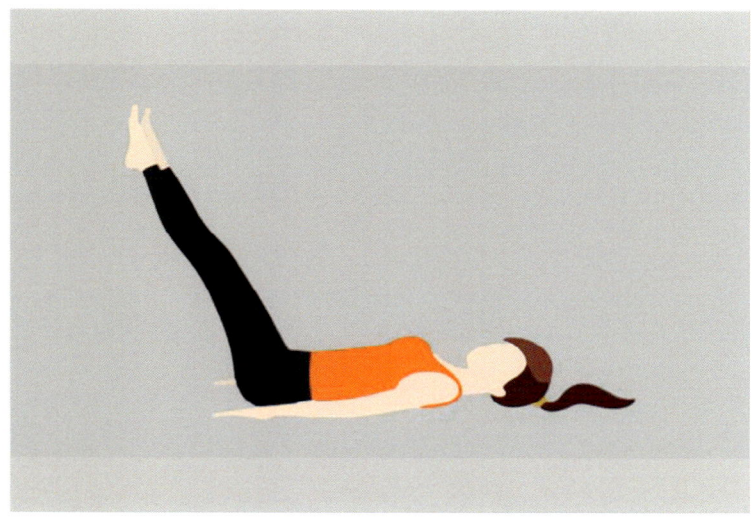

Illustration 4.11: Uttanpristh Aasan उत्तानपृष्ठआसन

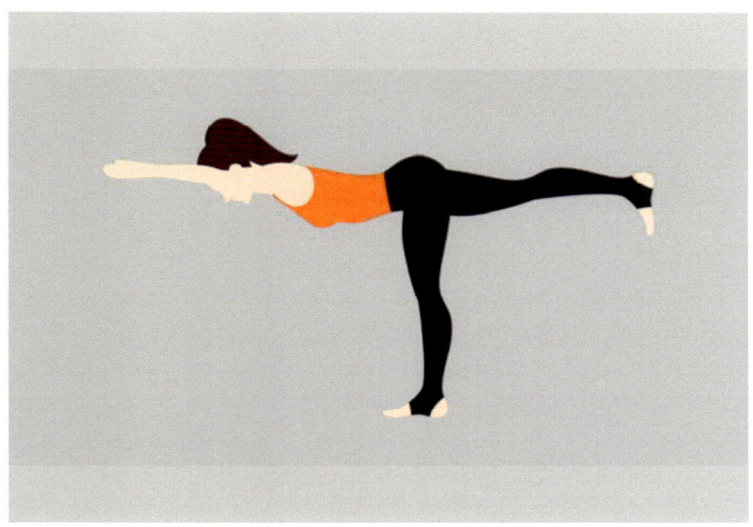

Illustration 4.12: Ekpaskot Aasan एकपसकोत

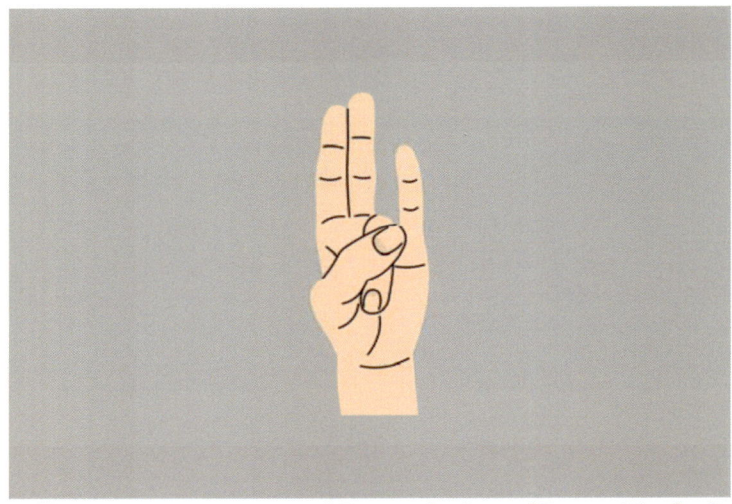

Illustration 4.13: Hand Formulations [Surya Mudra]

5

Anahata Chakra: The Confluence of Water, Earth, Fire, Air and Ether

The below-mentioned Vedic verse describes how kundalini will be moving through the anahata chakra अनाहत: चक्र, and what would be its traits and behaviour when it will be hosted there.

अत:धरपादनमसुसुमंख्या-लगनमध्वजाधोगडोर्ध्वमकत्यह-सोना-
पत्रमआधोवक्त्रमुद्हत-सुवर्णभावानेहवकर्दिसंतेरयुतमवेद:-वार्नर:!

We shall now discuss about the adhara lotus, which is attached to the mouth of the sushumna and is placed below the genitals and above the anus. It has four petals of crimson hue. Its head (mouth) hangs downwards and on the petals, are inscribed four letters from Va to Sa, of the shining colour of gold.

Anahata chakra अनाहत: चक्र is a Sanskrit connotation which in English would translate to, sound from one origin. It is worth mentioning that sound is normally created by contradicting behaviour of two things with one hitting and the other opposing. Like, when you clap, one hand is hitting the other hand whereby the other is trying to resist and hold on to its position or it can also be that both the hands are trying to hit and displace each other. The sound created from a particular origin when there is no contradictory stance or view or even engagement of the other, is anahata chakra अनाहत: चक्र. This is the chakra where your first introduction to "self" happens. It is here, where one discovers the difference and disparity between "my and self".

The name of this chakra signifies a state of freshness that unfolds, whereby a person is able to detach himself/herself and look at different and apparently contradictory experiences of life with a spirit of openness (expansion). Normally, we are not accustomed to the effect produced, following the confrontation of two opposite forces. Characteristically, in anahata chakra, there exists a possibility to integrate the two opposite forces and obtain the desired effect (sound, in this case), without any trigger of confrontation between the two. This energy is specific to cooperation and integration, which brings peace and a new perspective in a world which, so far up to this level (considering only the energies specific to the first three centres of force: mooldhara, manipura and swadishthana), was comprised of a more or less conscious confrontation between the opposite forces. The name anahata suggests, in fact, a synergetic effect of the interaction of energies at this level.

There are twelve petals which are inscribed with the following Sanskrit syllables:
1. Kam
2. Kham
3. Gam
4. Gham
5. Ngam
6. Cham
7. Chham
8. Jam
9. Jham
10. Nyam
11. Tam
12. Tham

The above syllables could be understood as corresponding to twelve divine qualities of the heart, namely:
1. Bliss
2. Peace
3. Harmony

4. Love
5. Understanding
6. Empathy
7. Clarity
8. Purity
9. Unity
10. Compassion
11. Kindness
12. Forgiveness

In common parlance, systems of understanding identify these divine qualities comparable to various reflexive modifications, away from the undifferentiated divine mind, with each one deemed as arising from the spiritual ignorance, viz.:

(a) Asha: wish, desire, hope
(b) Chinta: thoughtfulness, anxiety
(c) Cesta: effort
(d) Mamta: possessiveness, fondness
(e) Dhamba: arrogance, vanity
(f) Viveka: discrimination
(g) Vikalata: languor
(h) Ahamkara: conceit, egoism, pride
(i) Lolata: covetousness, avarice
(j) Kapata: duplicity, hypocrisy
(k) Vitarka: indecision, argumentativeness
(l) Anutapa: regret, burning misery

As per the Vedas, the sound created by this chakra is absolute in itself and has no recoiling, thereby meaning that there is no necessity for any rebound of the strike, for the sound to be sensed as complete. I would like to assert here, that in Sanskrit language, phonetics play a dominant role. Phonetics is basically musical/sound notes, which really do not have a meaning but definitely make and provide/extend "sense to the senses". For this very reason, we can safely presume why there cannot be a meaning attached to the "beej mantras", since they entail a sense which can only be experienced. In

Sanskrit, the energies are not driven by psychology (as when one is able to comprehend with the meaning of the things, corresponding emotions develop), but by those mantras which are a part of the real essence of the energies. My aim to highlight this subject matter was simply intended to avoid getting baffled by meanings in Google or the narratives extended by others. Rather, one should try and find out the meaning of the phonemes being mentioned as "chakra mantras", by experiencing the sense they transpire within. The role of the mantras and the way they should be recited would be duly addressed in another book.

Sound created by this chakra can be understood as the one generated, while clapping with a single hand. This is the sound which is complete and without any rebound. This is the chakra which germinates the consciousness to go beyond the five senses and experience life without having any defined "perspectives". As mentioned, it being non-contradictory in its virtue, this chakra also doesn't create taste, smell, and feel but by using this chakra in physical world, the sense of "touch" is what drives it. Quite confusing as it may sound, read each word again diligently and you would be able to derive the appropriate and correct conclusion and understand this chakra better before initiating the stimulations and the consequent activation of this chakra.

Anahata is associated with the ability to make decisions outside the realm of karma. In Manipura and below, a person is bound by the laws of karma and fate. In anahata, one makes decisions (by following one's heart"), based on one's higher self, and not by the unfulfilled emotions and desires of a lower nature. Accordingly, it is known as the heart chakra. It is also associated with love and compassion, charity towards others and psychic healing. Meditation in this chakra is known to bring about the following *siddhis* (abilities): one becomes a lord of speech, one is dear to women, one's presence controls the senses of others, and one can leave and enter the body at will.

Anahata Chakra: The Confluence of Water, Earth, Fire, Air...

Below anahata (at the solar plexus or sometimes on the near left side of the body), is a minor chakra known as hrit (or hriday, viz. "heart"), with eight petals. It has three regions, namely, a vermilion sun region, within which exists a white moon region, and further within which, is a deep-red fire region. Within this, exists a red wish-fulfilling tree, which symbolises the ability to manifest what one wishes to happen in the world.

Hrit chakra is sometimes also known as the surya (sun) chakra, which is located slightly to the left, below the heart. Its role is to absorb energy from the sun and provide heat to the body and other chakras (manipura in particular, to which it delivers the fire element).

The stimulations for this chakra are felt in and around the mid-rib area on the front side first and then post its establishment, the tingling sensations travel back to the lungs. When that happens and if you are observant enough, one would feel both sides of the chest in the mid-rib area, resonating with these tingling feelings and that too at a significant frequency and pitch. There are 12 major channels and 8 minor channels/tributaries which form part of this chakra and there are an equal number of openings through which the energy moves out and travels to other chakras and organs of the body. It is worth mentioning that for upward movement of the energy to take place, the next three chakras have to be mandatorily active, or else one won't be able to taste the essence of upward movement of the energy.

This chakra, apart from gains in the spiritual facet, also does contribute towards the societal life. The usage of words, the concepts, preferred companionship, the texture of tone, the sense of compassion, and the emotional quotient are some of the traits governed and guided by the energies of and from this chakra. This chakra encompasses the role of a power provider, responsible for balancing/regulating the flow of energy in all the chakras, provided they are activated. As such, the energy is not channeled in a unilateral direction, i.e. the energy is not only supposed to flow from the anahata chakra to other chakras, but is deemed the other way round also. The energy from the other chakras, especially from the lower three chakras (mentioned in the previous chapters), too moves upwards towards the heart chakra to blend. Anahata is said to be near to the heart. Due to its connection with touch (sense) and actions, it is associated with the skin and hands. In the endocrine system of the brain, anahata is said to be linked with the thalamus.

External and internal beauty, solace and comfort are the three major attributes necessary for an equitable functioning of this chakra. If one possesses these three virtues, there is a greater possibility that a person has already activated the anahata chakra, which is very much depicted in the yantra of this chakra too. Since this chakra is a confluence of air, water, earth, fire and ether, there is always a formation of newer shapes and designs. Thoughts of a person, performance scale of organs receiving, assimilating and transmitting the energy to and fro, flow of blood, oxygen richness of arteries and veins, are a few examples to understand the multi-faceted tasks this chakra engages in the domain of physical essence. The role of this chakra in the spiritual realm is mirrored by the contradictions in the behaviour of this chakra which are sublimed in a way that although one remains living but is yet non-contradictory. This component is better comprehended by experiencing it rather than relying on the theoretical aspect.

The basic and main sound from this chakra can be generated by holding the air in your heart, throat and under your tongue and then releasing it in the following order:
1) Tongue
2) Lungs
3) Throat

The above process is one of the methods for stimulating and activating this chakra. It shall be further illustrated in the mantra recitation segment in greater detail.

When this chakra gets activated, you would no longer be a prisoner of your own convictions but would rather be open to new learning and the ability to acquire and implement knowledge, which would be more experience-based than just being "hearsay". You would be clear in your thoughts and there won't be sacristy towards new things. You would be in possession of a reinvigorated memory and steer clear of distasteful experiences of the past. You will have a revitalized approach towards life and a more compassionate attitude towards others. You would be inclined towards the cosmic part of the universe, and there shall be an inclination to pursue what is not visible viz. "the energies". You would be poetic in your conversations and prefer to speak softly.

When dysfunctional, your traits would just be the opposite of what they should have been when anahata chakra is activated. You would be stubborn and adamant about your possessions. You would lack logic in your debates and even a little spark would prompt you to engage in a fight. You would easily succumb to arguments and physical altercations and intentionally like to suppress and harass people.

These manifestations apart, a dysfunctional anahata chakra also translates into physical inconveniences like stiff chest, stooping/bending of back while walking, curved-in and stiff/frozen shoulders. Mentally, an imbalanced heart chakra can result in issues such as co-dependence, manipulative behaviour, feeling of unworthiness, and inability to trust yourself or others.

The behavioral aspects of element air, in this chakra, can be classified into five different types of variations, namely:

(a) Praan Vaayu प्राणवायू: This can be understood as one which regulates and controls the organs and their functions.

(b) Vyaan Vaayu व्यानवायू: This can be inferred as one which imparts taste and flavours in life. Holistically, it may be conspicuous in relationships, or in our association with nature, or even in the basics of how and what we perceive about ourselves.

(c) Smaan Vaayu समानवायू: This can be implied as one defining the legitimacy of things by furnishing logics and keeping convictions at bay.

(d) Apaan Vaayu अपानवायू: This can be perceived as one which is responsible for the excretion of all types of "toxins" and waste from the body.

(e) Udaan Vayu उदानवायू: This can be understood as a form of air element responsible for regulation of heat. In other words, the maintenance and regulation of the water element in this chakra is ascertained by this aspect of element air.

Element air has two major variants—one that could be felt in the air around and the other that is present in the body. According to the Vedas, there are 49 such sub-types of air elements which are present in a human body. Irrespective of the age and size, the role of the above mentioned five variants can be broken down to 49 sub-types.

Mellowing down and softening of your stance, either psychologically or physically, furthers the possibility and provisions of bonding, may it be with an idea or with the energies. Simply putting, the feasibility exists if there is a "provision" of acceptability. There needs to be a harmonious integration between the heart chakra, the lower three chakras and the two chakras above. Sahastradhara chakra is independent of all these prerequisites and can only be activated once the 6 major chakras and 108 minor chakras are activated, to facilitate smooth movement of energy in all these chakras, whilst making its presence felt in the anahata chakra.

Before you decide on to adopt the accepted measures to stimulate and initiate the process of activating the anahata chakra, the following methodology should be adhered to:

(a) Sit in a quiet and comfortable position in a dim lit room, where deep inhaling and exhaling could be managed.

(b) When you have inhaled sufficiently, protrude your chest outwards and hold onto the position for as long as you can.

(c) While holding onto this position of chest protruding out, try to squeeze your belly inside, in order to create a striking difference between the chest and the abdomen.
(d) Continuing with the position outlined in (c), lift your shoulders upwards and then pull them down immediately in a shoulder shrugging manner.
(e) Try and get a sense of the enhanced heart beat while maintaining your focus on the same.
(f) Feel the sensations in your body, while upholding the position mentioned in points (b) and (c).
(g) Feel the varying temperatures in your lower chakras; the mooldhara chakra should be heated or warm, while the swadishthana chakra would be cold and the manipura chakra would be resonating with varying degree of heat and cold temperatures. If these attributes are lacking, repeat the procedure from (a) to (d).
(h) Exhale and repeat this exercise for at least 8-10 times for the anahata chakra and stimulation of the lower three chakras before commencing the yog aasan associated with this chakra.

For the stimulation and activation of this chakra, control over "breath" is quite crucial. Breathing is the only activity which defines all of us as living. For this chakra, breath would be the focal point. How deep can one inhale and the duration of exhaling are the defining factors for this chakra. Inhalation of oxygen provides energy to the body and the organs to function properly. Greater the inhalation, greater would be the supply of oxygen to these organs. Comparatively, when we exhale, we are downsizing stress. Resultantly, longer is the exhaling process, greater would be the stress released. Therefore, keep your focus on breath, as this would be the key to accomplish the endeavour of activating the anahata chakra.

Breathing स्वाँस

For this chakra, breath is the most crucial and important factor. It would be the breathing patterns which will determine the course of activating this chakra. To start with, establish a comfortable position. I would advise against sitting on a bed or on a soft mattress in order to ensure an erect back. Instead, you can choose to sit on a sofa or a chair if sitting on the floor is cumbersome. Now, inhale softly but deeply and continue with the same till you hit the limit of bending your back or sensing some imbalance. Secure the breath in your lungs, and try to push the inhaled air from the front part of your lungs to the back part. At this point, while attempting to exhale, take the breath to the tip of the nostrils (don't let it go out) and then suck it in to the back of lungs. Repeat this exercise as per your comfort zone. Before slowly letting the air exhale, repeat the process for around 30-50 times (depending upon the capacity of your lungs). More importantly, before attempting this exercise, duly consult a doctor about your physical status and only contemplate engaging into it, post the approval and consent of your doctor.

Physical Yog योग

Chakra Swas Aasan चक्रस्वाँसआसन

We shall start with a very basic and easy exercise. Position yourself in sidh aasan सिद्धआसन or padma aasan पद्माआसन with bent elbows, and hands resting/fingers touching the shoulder. While in this position, inhale deeply and hold the breath in your lungs. To exhale, push the air out of your lungs whilst straightening your hands upwards. Repeat this exercise for at least 20-40 times, without resting in between. This exercise shall stimulate your anahata chakra while extending stimulations to your mooldhara chakra too.

(Refer to Illustration 5.1: **Chakra Swas Aasan** चक्रस्वाँसआसन *at Page No. 113)*

Yog Mudra योगमुद्रा

For performing this aasan, you need to stand straight with an erect back. Now, stretch your legs just a little apart sideways. From this position, try and clasp fingers of both the hands at the back. Hold this position for a while and then in that clasped state of fingers, try and move your hands away from the body, corresponding with the forward bending of your body till the time your upper torso is almost perpendicular to the ground below. Hold onto this position as per your comfort levels without feeling breathless. Return to the original position of standing straight with legs a bit apart from each other. Repeat this exercise for at least 30 times before moving onto the next exercise. This exercise would help in release of stress in the chest area, shoulders, back, and the cervical and neck area, apart from providing ease in breathing, which as mentioned above, is one of the most crucial components for activating the anahata chakra.

(Refer to Illustration 5.2: **Yog Mudra** योगमुद्रा *at Page No. 113)*

Gaumukh Aasan गौमुखआसन

For performing this aasan, you need to stand straight on a firm ground with your feet at a comfortable distance from each other. Now, bend your right hand and the portion of the hand which is below the elbow. Move it towards the back of your chest in the bent arm position and try touching it with your neck or shoulders from the back. When this posture is attained, raise your left hand and bend it in such a way that fingers of the left hand should clap with those of the right hand. Hold it as long as you are comfortable without stretching dangerously, to avoid damage to the neck and cervical muscles. Return to the normal standing position with hands at the side of your body. Repeat this exercise with the left hand in the back position and right hand clasping it. Rerun this exercise for at least 30-60 times with the period of holding the clasped hands nothing less than 60-80 seconds.

(Refer to Illustration 5.3: **Gaumukh Aasan** गौमुखआसन *at Page No. 114)*

Parig Aasan प्रिगआसन

For performing this aasan, stand straight with your legs comfortably placed sideways and stretched apart. Now, bend your right knee and sit on the bent right leg while keeping your left leg stretched, resting on its heel. Even as you maintain this position, with your right hand, try touching the ground around the calf muscle of your bent right leg while keeping your left hand fully stretched over the head. Now, bend backwards while keeping your eyes on the spread out fingers of your left hand. Make an effort to hold onto this position for a convenient time period, without feeling breathless. Return to the original position of standing, with legs comfortably stretched apart. Repeat this exercise with the other leg, allowing the same duration. It is strongly recommended to solicit a doctor's advice before undertaking the above exercise or any other for that matter.

*(Refer to Illustration 5.4: **Parig Aasan** प्रिगआसन at Page No. 114)*

Mtsaya Aasan मत्स्यआसन

To carry out this aasan, lie down on your back with your hands comfortably resting around the waist area. Now, try and bend your head inwards so that your chest and shoulders are slightly lifted from the floor while keeping your hands on the ground. Try to accommodate the entire load of chest and shoulders on your neck area with no assistance from arms. Maintain this position for as long as you can, without inviting any strain on the neck, back, and cervical area. It is essential not to hold the stretched position while feeling breathless, ensuring that breathing remains normal.

*(Refer to Illustration 5.5: **Mtsaya Aasan** मत्स्यआसन at Page No. 115)*

Ustr Aasan उत्रआसन

For performing this aasan, sit on the bent knees whilst keeping your spine erect and shoulders comfortably spread and the chest area protruding out. Now place your hands on the waist, and push the chest further in front while bending your spine backwards. The degree of bending the spine is entirely dependent on your flexibility levels. Further, touch the heels of the feet with your hands and maintain this position for a significant period. Under no circumstances, try and overdo, as it may prove detrimental for the back.

(Refer to Illustration 5.6: **Ustr Aasan** उस्त्रआसन *at Page No. 115)*

Bhujang Aasan भुजंगआसन

For performing this aasan, lie down on your belly and bring your folded arms close to your chest and using the strength of your arms with the support of spine muscles, lift your upper torso from the ground while keeping your pelvis and lower torso on the ground. Now, lift your body and stretch backwards while keeping the maximum weight on the arms, which would be almost straight by now. Remain in this position as per your comforting levels and slowly return to the position of lying on your belly.

(Refer to Illustration 5.7: **Bhujang Aasan** भुजंगआसन *at Page No. 116)*

Adho Mukhvkr Aasan आदोमुख्क्रआसन

For realizing this aasan, you would require a table or have to stand next to a wall. Stand straight with your legs comfortably placed apart. Bend forward and try to touch the ground in front of you with your palms. Hold onto this position, and place your right foot on the table and lift your left leg and accordingly place it on the table (if you choose to do it against the wall, then lift your right leg and place your foot firmly and completely against the wall and raise your left leg adjacent to the right leg). Preferably, the height of the table should be close to your waist length. Initially, you may choose to keep the height lower and try and balance your weight on your legs and arms. Try maintaining this position for a comfortable duration while simultaneously balancing your weight. You can now slowly return to the standing position before repeating the exercise. The advanced version of this exercise is sheesh aasan शीषआसन, which should only be attempted under an expert supervision.

(Refer to Illustration 5.8: **Adho Mukhvkr Aasan** आदोमुख्क्रआसन *at Page No. 116)*

Urdv Dhanur Aasan ऊर्ध्वधनुरआसन

To perform this aasan, you need to lie on your back and bend the knees one by one. While sticking to this position, lift your right hand and bend it in a way that the palm of the right hand rests near the back of the right shoulder. Repeat the same with the other hand also.

Now, try and lift your chest, shoulders and belly on your arms while letting your pelvis weight supported by the legs. Try and push your belly outwards while maintaining the stretched posture. Pursue this exercise only after duly consulting your doctor.

(Refer to Illustration 5.9: **Urdv Dhanur Aasan** ऊर्ध्वधनुरआसन *at Page No. 117)*

Hand Formulations बंध

Since anahata chakra is the one responsible for governing the emotions, and their generation and interpretation, there can be no discounting the fact that all what is "life" are just emotions. It is these emotions which have been a driving force—even while you are browsing through this book to stimulate and activate your chakras for making your life better than what is now, is a manifestation of these emotions.

The hand formulations बंध for this chakra is denominated as rudra mudra रुद्रमुद्रा. To form this mudra, join the tips of your thumb, index finger and the ring finger. As this formulation is effectual in stimulating the three elements viz. earth, ether and fire, only forming the mudra won't suffice. One needs to be observant about the changes, consequential upon forming this mudra.

One should be able to sense the variation in temperature in all the three fingers, namely, thumb, index, and the ring finger. If you are benumbed of the senses so generated, you need to refocus in a righteous manner.

(Refer to Illustration 5.10: **Hand Formulations** [Rudra Mudra] *at Page No. 117)*

Focus-based Exercises ध्यानक्रिया

These exercises entail your complete attention on the mid-rib point of chest area. Do not get distracted when you start feeling the tingling stimulations in that area. Let the tingling sensations persist while you focus on the mid-rib point area of chest and feel the rise and fall in temperature.

Mantras Recitation मंत्रउच्चारण

The mantra for the anahata chakra is

YAYAYAYAYAAMAMAMAMAMYAMYAMYAM

During the recitation of this mantra, one would be biologically tempted to exhale. However, try to inhale during the recitation of the correct texture. As outlined in the Vedas, and also experienced otherwise, the best results are obtained when recited while inhaling.

This mantra has proven effective in curing several psychological ailments also. Undoubtedly, there are variations which need to be incorporated, and presumably, the best results are achieved, if done under an expert supervision.

Naad Kriya ध्वनीयोग

To be able to hear and sense the movement of energy in the anahata chakra, sit in a relaxed posture (avoid sitting on a bed). You may choose to close your eyes if you concentration levels are not too high and you get distracted by the sight/vision sense. Now, focus on the end part of your rib cage and hear the movement of energy travelling inward and outward because of the anahata chakra. Keep your concentration stable and hear the movement. You may hear certain rumbling sounds initially and after sometime, these sounds would change into that of a gong, or a chime (depending upon what is the activation level of your lower three chakras).

Yantra Sadhna यंत्रसाधना

This yantra of root chakra is formed by positioning the body (using hands/arms, legs) in such a way that when you breathe, the stimulations caused by the usual posture of the body occur at the root chakra. For root chakra, twist your legs in such a way that they entangle/grope each other while standing and repeat the same for the arms too with a subtle difference, that at the end of the groping of arms, the palms of the hands face each other.

Hold onto this position while breathing normally, till the time you are comfortable. Now, gently entangle your arms and legs, and relax by engaging into normal stretching exercises and then repeat it again. It is desired that your total holding period for this formulation should be at least 20 minutes (inclusive of the repetitions) initially, and it may further be increased as per your strength and endurance.

Tantra Sadhna तंत्रसाधना

This facet of the chakra meditation is beyond the ambit of this book.

Illustrative Representation of Aasana's

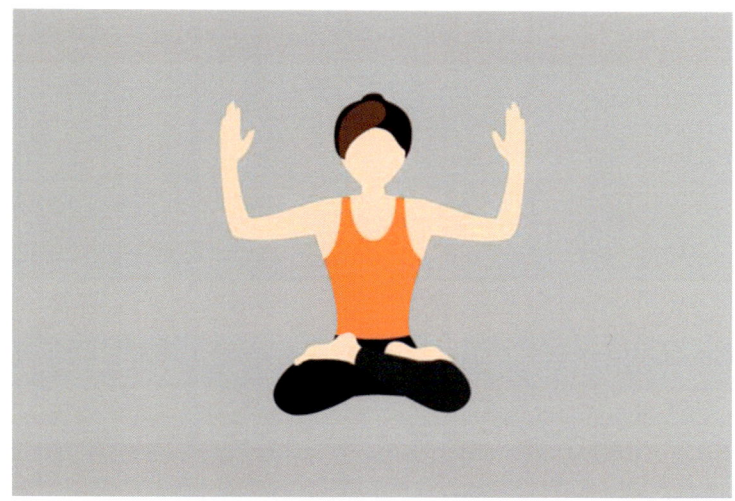

Illustration 5.1: Chakra Swas Aasan चक्रस्वाँसआसन

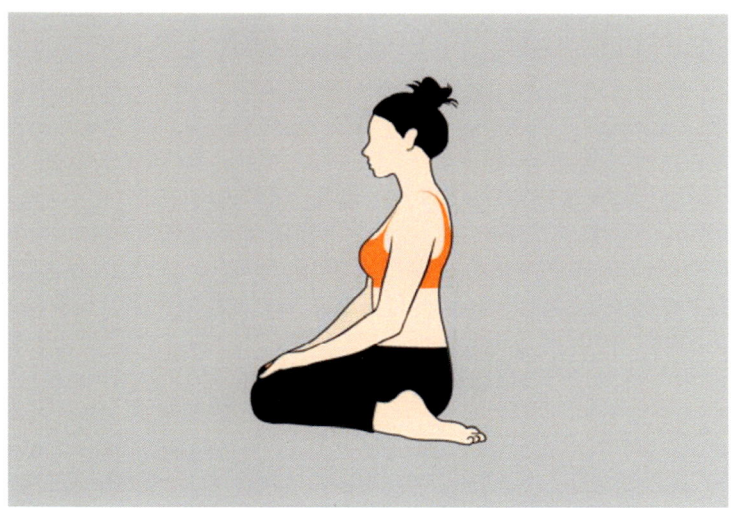

Illustration 5.2: Yog Mudra योगमुद्रा

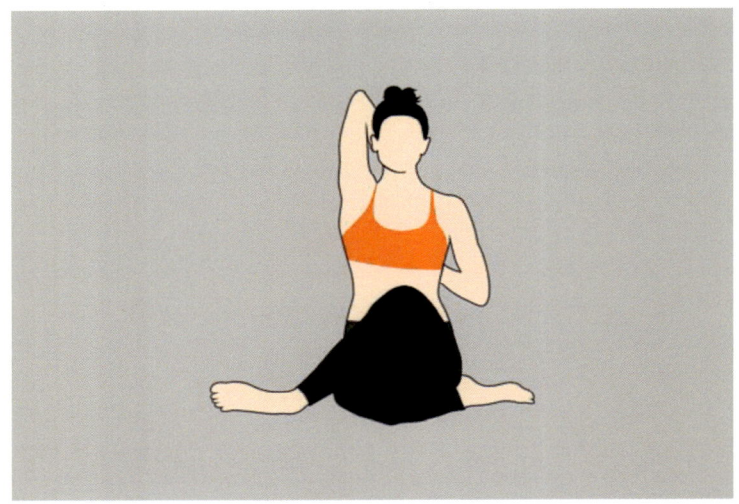

Illustration 5.3: Gaumukh Aasan गौमुखआसन

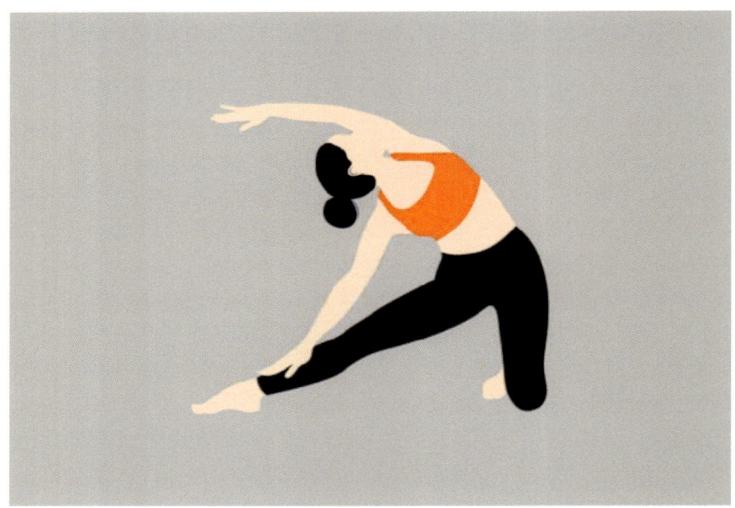

Illustration 5.4: Parig Aasan प्रिगआसन

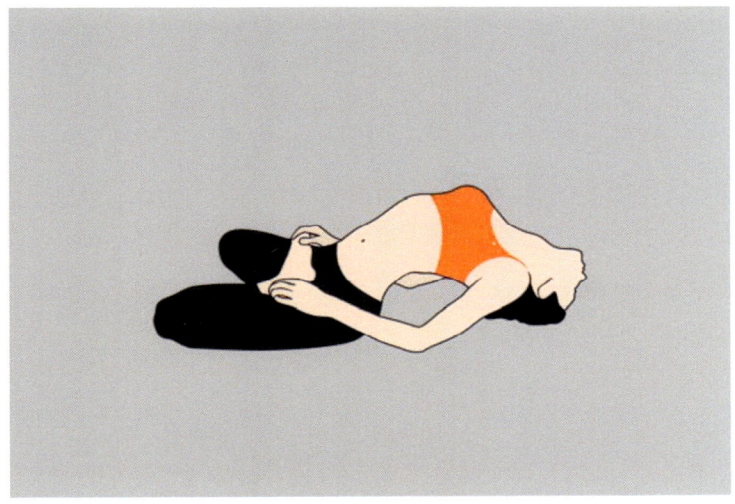

Illustration 5.5: Mtsaya Aasan मत्स्यआसन

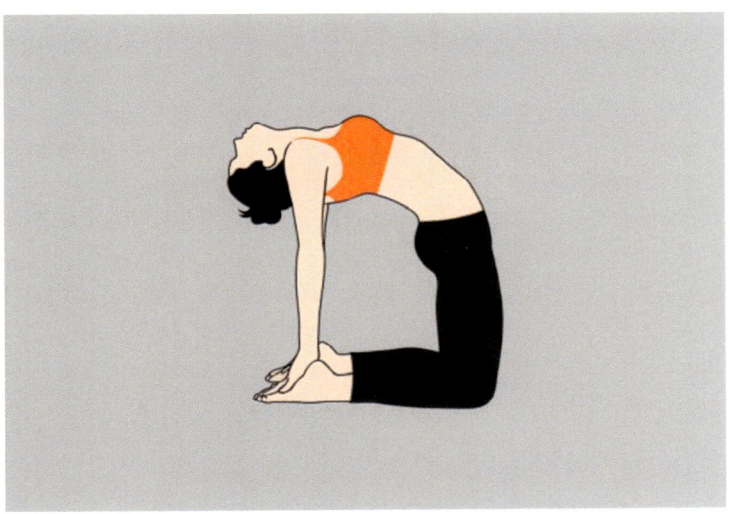

Illustration 5.6: Ustr Aasan उस्त्रआसन

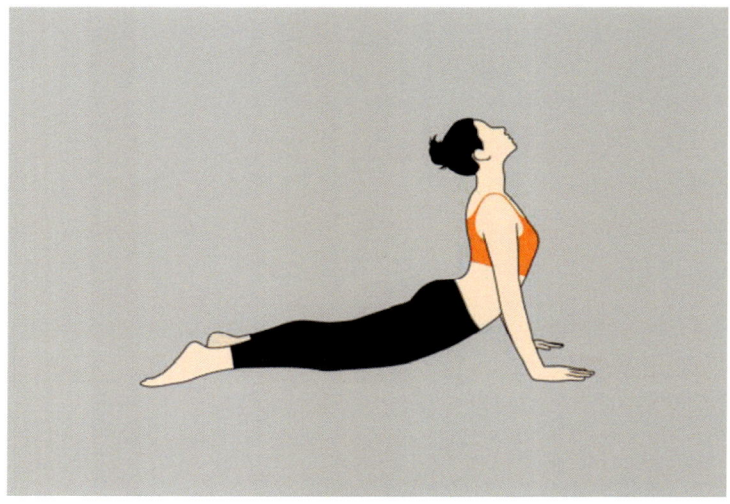

Illustration 5.7: Bhujang Aasan भुजंगआसन

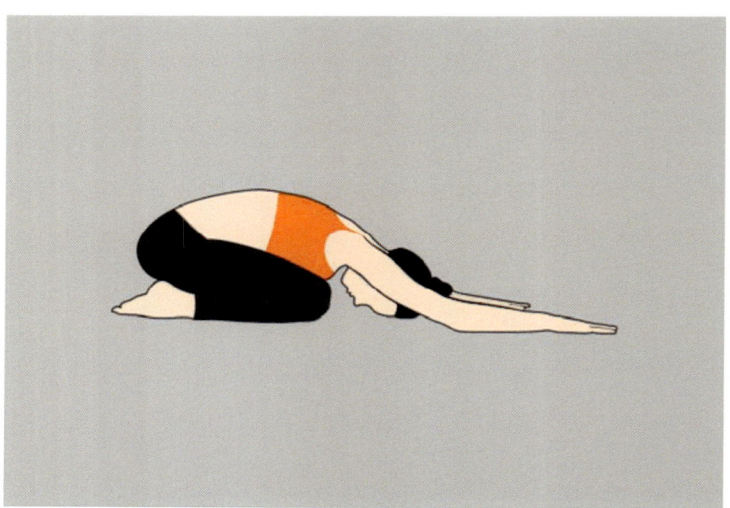

Illustration 5.8: Adho Mukhvkr Aasan आदोमुख्क्क्रआसन

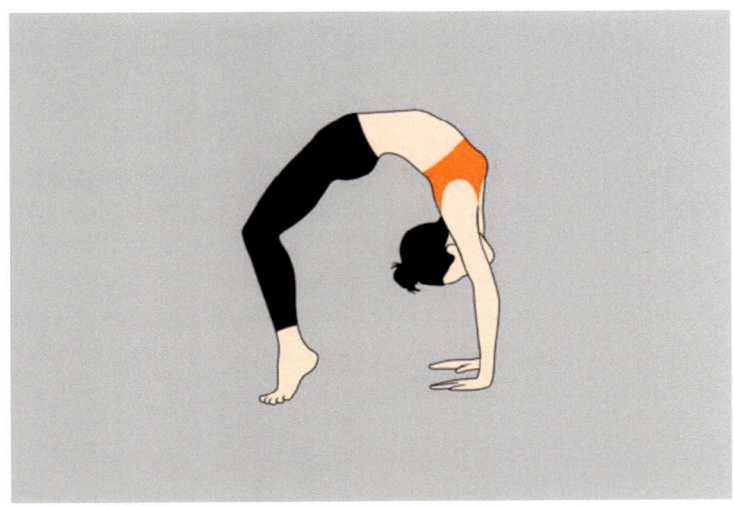

Illustration 5.9: Urdv Dhanur Aasan ऊर्ध्वधनुरआसन

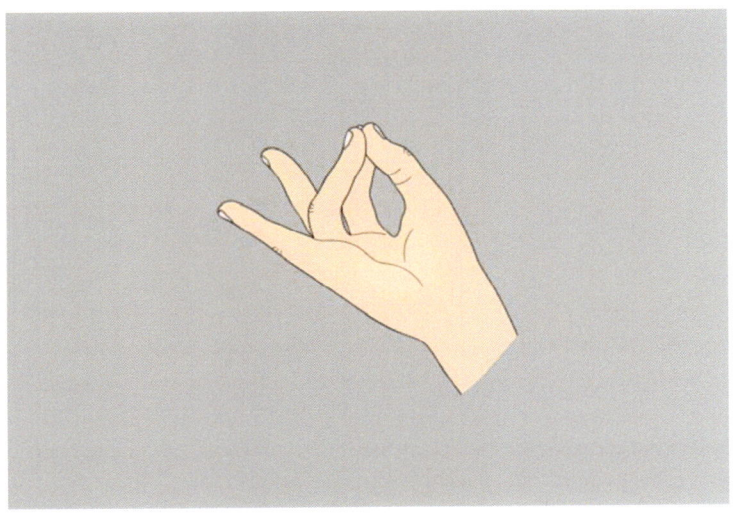

Illustration 5.10: Hand Formulations [Rudra Mudra]

6

Vishudhi Chakra: Ether

This chakra assumes significance wherein one can assume to have taken the first step of traversing into the cosmic energy. In other words, an individual can employ the behavioral aspects of this chakra in spiritual world—the world which is beyond comprehensive emotions and energy being the "sole" and the "soul" being the only carrier.

अमूसिमध्ग्ययसकटुसकोणसक्रमसम्बूध्भासीसुलसटाकौरवऋहृटतत्ल्स्तपितावर्णमत
ड़ितकोमलअंगमतडान्तेसमस्तेधैर्य: सव:बिजम

The lotus is the square region of prithvi, surrounded by eight lustrous spears. It is of shining yellow colour and appears magnificent like lightening.

This chakra is around the throat area—not exactly in the throat—but in the region where the chest starts specifically in between the two cartilages, supporting the neck from the front side. The sensations in this chakra would only be manifest on the front side. As and when they occur, one would be able to feel how they travel all over the throat area. A discernible change can be witnessed in the speaking tone, post these sensations, following the activation of this chakra.

In accordance with the Vedic traditions, this chakra can be described as having a "white colour", with sixteen "purple" or "smoke-coloured petals". Within the pericarp, is a sky blue triangle pointed in a downward position, depicting a white region in a circular shape, representational of a full moon. This characterizes the element of akasha or "ether". This region is represented by the deity Ambara, which is also white in colour and is depicted by four arms, holding a noose and a goad. The deity Ambara makes gestures of granting boons and dispelling fear while seated upon a white elephant. The silver crescent is the lunar symbol of nada—the pure cosmic sound. The crescent is symbolic of purity, and purification is a vital aspect of vishudhi chakra.

There are 16 nerves नाड़ी, which confluence to circulate the energy outwards from the above one chakra and below one chakra—as anahata chakra, post the assimilation of the energy from the lower three chakras, converts the energy into a different form. These 16 nerves नाड़ी tend to remain active, but are influenced by any emotional or psychological stress, and/or excessive thinking or talking, possibly resulting in deviation in course. However, it may not be necessarily in a dormant state in all individuals; perhaps the chosen ones are blessed to have these nerves नाड़ी in an active state. Due to these active nerves नाड़ी, an individual is able to realise the non-functioning of the chakras and aspires to activate them. Interestingly, this possibility is what has precisely has led you to glance through this book.

As outlined above, these 16 nerves नाड़ी, communicate with the chakra by bringing in the energy and transferring the same from the chakra to the other organs. If the agya chakra आज्ञाचक्र is active, it is also a beneficiary, else the energy from this chakra or for that matter from any other chakra, would remain below the neck area only.

The dominant element for this chakra is ether, with fire, earth, water, and air, present in small ratios. Nonetheless, their significance cannot be undermined by their sheer volumes. Rather, it is their contribution towards the formation of shape, texture and nature of energy, which is a critical factor. Ether element won't be able to transfer the energy in itself if there is no support from element earth. Correspondingly, element earth in turn cannot help in itself if it is not assisted by element fire and furthermore element fire cannot be there without any facilitation extended by element air. Hence, inter-dependence of all the elements is integral for the chakra(s) to function, and curing of a chakra can be one of the methods to correct any element deficiency. The alternate method could be rectify the elements and hence cure the chakras. Whatsoever method one may choose to adopt, the results should be evident, and there is no role or scope of any belief or faith, at least not in the Vedic system of things.

Vishudhi chakra is located in the neck area and throat. Due to its association with hearing and speaking, it is related to ears and mouth respectively.

Vishudhi is often linked with the thyroid gland in the human endocrine system. This gland is in the neck, and produces hormones essential for growth and maturation. Excessive stress, namely fear and fear of speaking out, are said to affect the throat chakra, and as a consequence, thyroid problems arise. Singing is a harmless and beneficial way of stimulating the throat chakra, whereas rubbing or hitting of the throat area can prove to be harmful.

Vishudhi chakra is also acknowledged as a purification center, where the nectar *amrita* drips down from the bindu chakra and splits into a pure and a poison form. In its most abstract form, it is associated with higher discrimination and also associated with creativity and self-expression. It is believed that when vishudhi is blocked, a person undergoes decay and death. Simultaneously, when it is open, negative experiences get transformed into wisdom and learning. The success and failure in an individual's life are said to depend upon the state of this chakra—whether it is polluted or is clean. The feeling of being guilty is stated as the most prominent reason for this chakra to block the kundalini energy from moving upwards.

Meditation within the ambit of this chakra is supposed to induce various *siddhis* of occult powers, viz. vision of the three periods—past, present and future; freedom from disease and old age; elimination of danger; and the ability to move the three worlds.

Vishudhi chakra incorporates five dimensions in its virtue and traits. Five major outcomes that can be achieved, post activation of this chakra are:
1. A person becomes poetic in his/her conduct and appreciates things around.
2. A person comprehends with things well and "language" isn't the only recourse for such a person to conceive things.
3. A person acknowledges and recognises "solace" and tends to remain in that "undisturbed" state of mind, perpetually.
4. A person maintains greater immunity.
5. A person does not feel "perturbed or lost" if struck by a sorrow or grief.

The literal connotation of the word "vishudhi" means, without any boundaries. It can also be implied in the sense of a person having no restrains or restrictions, following the activation of vishudhi chakra. An explicit reasoning for this could be that a person has won over all the emotions and other restrictive traits—things which may be/would be/will be restricting a person to achieve as to what he/she desires.

Closely related to vishudhi chakra is a minor chakra, located in the roof of the mouth and termed as lalana/taalu. It is described as possessing 12 red or white petals that correspond to the virtues of respect, contentment, offence, self-control, pride, affection, sorrow, depression, purity, dissatisfaction, honour and anxiety. Inside, there is a moon region which is circular in nature and red in colour that acts as a reservoir for the nectar (amrit). When vishudhi is inactive, this nectar runs downwards into the manipura and consumed thereupon, resulting in physical degeneration. Through practices such as khechari mudra, the nectar can be made to enter vishudhi, where it is purified, and eventually becomes a nectar of immortality.

Post-activation of this chakra, there is a feeling of intoxication, which may prevail. One would be placed in a different zone, quite similar to what people experience post having liquor. Intrigued by the subject, the remaining "dressing up" would appear trivial and a waste.

This is one of those chakras where mantra recitation proves more efficient than the physical yog. However, this statement does not undermine the relevance of physical yog for this chakra. This is so because, there is only one chakra beyond this chakra, which has provisions to be stimulated by physical yog, since the ratio of space and ether in a physical body is trivial in a "solitary" aspect.

The mantra for this chakra is inspired by the notes of music, generated by the 16 nerves नाड़ी. There are 14 ways through which a mantra can be recited for this chakra or for that matter, recitation of the mantra for any reason or cause. These are:

1. Nitya Jap नित्यजप: Recitation which is done on a daily basis and in fixed count.
2. Nimaitik Jap नेमैतिकजप: Recitation which remains within and even if one isn't willingly reciting, the mantra can be heard from inside.
3. Kaamya Jap काम्यजप: Recitation done for a special cause.
4. Nishid Jap निषिद्धजप: Recitation which isn't time restricted.
5. Paraishchit Jap प्राईषचितजप: Recitation in specific numbers, conducted as an act on penance.
6. Achal Jap अचलजप: Recitation which is accomplished under strict principles and procedures.
7. Chal Jap चलजप: Recitation which isn't bound by place, occasion or numbers.
8. Vaachik Jap वाचिकजप: Recitation which is spoken loud.
9. Apanchchu Jap अपाँचुजप: Recitation not restricted to a specific number than what has been prescribed.

10. Bharamar Jap भ्रमरजप: Recitation in which the body temperature is made to rise—supposedly, one of the most intense ones.
11. Maanas Jap मानसजप: Recitation which is discharged at all times, irrespective of the act.
12. Akhand Jap अखंडजप: Recitation which is done for a special cause and all the principles and procedures are strictly adhered to.
13. Ajapa Jap अजपाजप: Recitation which is independent of any number count and can be started or ended as per wish.
14. Prdikshna Jap पर्दिक्शनजप: Recitation which is result-oriented—normally, this procedure is applied for balancing the elements.

While submitting to vishudhi chakra, one would taste the sense and experience of "life energies", labeled as pran प्राण in the Sanskrit language. The functioning of pran प्राण is primal in constituting living, and the recognition of this movement is our realization of being alive. Without any explicit correlation, the presence and movement of pran प्राण is the defining principle of endorsing "awareness" (a thing which is quite popular but isn't widely "experienced").

It is this awareness, which brings to the fore, the movements of energy and also the blockades. As previously mentioned, stress and other emotional facets lead to creating blockages in the nerves which primarily act as conduit for the transfer of energy. Even if you do not desire and are mindful of not letting the "external-motions" (popularly known as emotions) affect you or stay with you as part of your cognitive memory, still there is a residual which would stick with you, till the time they are vented. The scenario is quite distinguishable for people who are "emotional" to each and everything in their life, especially with regards to their "dear ones". Inarguably, it would be more challenging for such people to get off those effects from their system—biological or psychological. To elaborate, whatsoever you speak or hear, does not only remain confined to the ears or throat, rather it travels across the body. Since each and every word has an inherent specific vibration, the resonance travels across the system. Even while reading this book, there are vibrations travelling within your system, while you speak to yourself. Bearing this in mind, specific names have been designated to gods, and people are encouraged to recite/spell out those names, as these names have been conceptualised and designed in a manner through which specific vibrations, at a defined frequency, travels within the body. In Vedic system, sound has four major styles. These are, namely:

1. Praa परा: The one beyond the mass and the matter.
2. Pashynti पश्यन्ति: The one which defines the mass and the matter (what a physical body is made up of).
3. Madhyma मध्यमा: The sound which is/should be used for reciting the mantras; not audible from outside.
4. Vaikri वैक्रि: The common sound; like what you can hear even while reading this.

Breathing स्वाँस

In order to cure and stimulate your vishudhi chakra, one need to regulate the breath in a manner, that inhaling and exhaling is carried out in small amounts. Expressly, inhale very slowly and stop and hold onto the inhaled breath. Further, inhale again and pause while holding the breath inside and resume inhaling again. When you feel you cannot hold it any longer, exhale in small proportions and stop, holding the rest of the air inside you. Now, exhale again whilst holding the remaining breath inside. Repeat the process till you exhale fully. One would yield better results if the quantum of intervals while inhaling and exhaling is larger. However, this does not discount the fact that one needs to duly consult a doctor before attempting to accomplish this exercise.

Physical Yog योग

There are not many a physical योग which can directly assist in stimulating this chakra. Nonetheless, the ones which are significant in stimulating the right chord and at a right frequency are mentioned.

Jallandhar Bandh Yog जालंधरबंधयोग

For performing this yog, one may choose to sit in a sidh aasan सिद्धआसन or a padma aasan पद्माआसन while keeping the back erect. While this posture is established, you need to inhale (quantity of the inhaled breath should be a bit more than the usual), and bend your neck in such a manner so as to touch the collar bone with your chin, while maintaining the back to be in an erect position. Maintain this position whilst holding onto your breath, as long as you are comfortable with. Now, slowly pull back your neck to the normal position while exhaling. Do ensure that the exhaling and lifting up of the neck should be synchronization to ascertain the entirety of exhalation.

(Refer to Illustration 6.1: **Jallandhar Bandh Yog** जालंधरबंधयोग *at Page No. 132)*

Setu Bandh Sarvang Aasan सेतुबंधसर्वांगआसन

In this aasan, you need to lie down on your back, with legs stretched forward. Now, bend your knees and lift your pelvis area while keeping your shoulders and head on the ground. Hold onto this position and bring your arms into the space, created by lifting up of your lower torso and let the hands clip together. Hold this position as per your comfort zone, and when you choose to return, first untangle the hands and then by moving your arms to the side of the body, gently let your body touch the ground. As your torso has touched the ground slowly, stretch your legs forward and relax before repeating the exercise.

(Refer to Illustration 6.2: **Setu Bandh Sarvang Aasan** सेतुबंधसर्वांगआसन *at Page No. 132)*

Mtsaya Aasan मत्स्यआसन

For executing this aasan, lie down on your back with hands resting comfortably, around the waist area. Now, try and bend your head inwards in such a fashion that your chest and shoulders could be slightly lifted from the floor while keeping the hands on ground. Try to have the entire load of the chest and shoulders on your neck without any assistance from the arms. Preferably, maintain this position for as long as you can, and at no instance, strain your neck, back, and cervical area. Additionally, do not hold the stretched position in case breathlessness is felt.

(Refer to Illustration 6.3: **Mtsaya Aasan** मत्स्यआसन *at Page No. 133)*

Trikon Aasan त्रिकोणआसन

To carry out this aasan, stand straight with an erect back. Stretch your legs sideways in a position you are comfortable holding while able to balance yourself. While in this position, move your right arm towards the back of your right leg in a manner that you are able to hold the heel of your right leg. Move your left arm over your head and position your head in a posture that projects as if you are following your left arm and able to see the fingers of your left hand. Hold onto this position while maintaining the breath. Stick to the position as per your comfort levels before returning to the standing pose, with legs stretched sideways. Relax and breathe normally, before repeating the exercise on the other side. This aasan is known to improve digestion and provides relief from stiff legs and hips and has also been found beneficial in healing sciatica pain.

(Refer to Illustration 6.4: **Trikon Aasan** त्रिकोणआसन *at Page No. 133)*

Parivrata Prasarvkon Aasan परिवृत्त पर्सर्वकोणआसन

For performing this aasan, stand straight with an erect back. Now, stretch your legs sideways in a comfortable position and bend your right knee with your right hand on the ground. From the backside of the right foot, stretch your left hand over your head in a manner which enables you to touch the ground. Avoid extensive stretching to brush off any injuries. Hold onto this position as long as you are comfortable while managing normal breathing. Going forward, return to the standing position and relax for a while. Repeat the exercise on the other side also. This aasana extends strength to the shoulders and collar bone area and enhances chest strength.

(Refer to Illustration 6.5: **Parivrata Prasarvkon Aasan** परिवृत्त पर्सर्वकोणआसन *at Page No. 134)*

Ardh Chandra Aasan अर्धचंद्रआसन

To realize this aasan, stand straight with an erect back and stretching the legs sideways. From this position, turn your torso towards the right side with a bent right knee and left leg almost stretched. Now from this position, bend your back forward and try touching the ground on your right side with a similar face angle. Hold onto this position as per the comfort levels while ensuring no breathlessness. Now, return to the position where you are standing with legs stretched sideways and relax for a while. Repeat the exercise on the other side too.

(Refer to Illustration 6.6: **Ardh Chandra Aasan** अर्धचंद्रआसन *at Page No. 134)*

Viprit Virbhadar Aasan विप्रीतवीरभद्रआसन

For performing this aasan, stand straight with an erect back. Following this position, stretch your legs sideways till you are comfortable maintaining the same. Now, turn your torso towards the right leg and raise your right hand above your head while keeping your left hand on the thighs or knees of straight and stretched left leg and the bent right knee. Allow your head to follow your hand, bending it a little backwards, as if to watch the fingers of the right hand. Hold onto this position while maintaining heavy and hard breathing. While retaining the position in conformity with the comfort level, return to the position of stretched legs while keeping the torso straight. Relax, before doing this exercise on the other side. This aasana has been rewarding in providing strength to the legs, abdominal area and shoulders, in addition to dispensing flexibility.

(Refer to Illustration 6.7: **Viprit Virbhadar Aasan** विप्रीतवीरभद्रआसन *at Page No. 135)*

Yog Mudra योगमुद्रा

For performing this aasan, stand straight with an erect back. Now, stretch your legs just a little apart sideways. From this position, clasp the fingers of your hands from the back. Maintain this position for a while and fingers being in a clasped state, try moving your hands away from the body, corresponding with the forward bending of your body till the time the upper torso is almost in a perpendicular position to the ground below. While ensuring that you do not experience breathlessness, return to the original position of standing straight, with legs a bit away from each other. Repeat this exercise for at least 30 times before moving onto the next exercise. This exercise shall help you release stress in your chest area, shoulders, back, cervical and the neck area, apart from easing the breathing.

(Refer to Illustration 6.8: **Yog Mudra** योगमुद्रा *at Page No. 135)*

Parig Aasan प्रिगआसन

To carry out this aasan, stand straight with your legs comfortably stretched apart sideways. Bend your right knee and sit on your bent right leg whilst keeping your left leg stretched, resting on its heel. Whilst maintaining this position, with your right hand, try touching the ground around the calf muscle of your bent right leg while keeping your left hand fully stretched over your head. Now, bend backwards while keeping your eyes on the spread out fingers of your left hand. Try holding this position as long as you are comfortable and not feeling breathless. Return to the original position of standing with legs comfortably stretched apart. Rerun this exercise with the other leg also, keeping intact the time frame.

It is strongly recommended to consult a doctor before attempting the above or any other exercise for that matter.

(Refer to Illustration 6.9: **Parig Aasan** प्रिगआसन *at Page No. 136)*

Gaumukh Aasan गौमुखआसन

To execute this aasan, stand straight on a firm ground with your feet at a comfortable distance from each other. Now, bend your right hand and the portion of the hand which is below the elbow and move it towards the back of your chest in the bent arm position, touching the neck or shoulders from the back. While in this position, raise your left hand and bend it in a way that the fingers of the left hand clasp with those of the right hand. Keep yourself positioned to the best possible ease and avoid any dangerous stretching which may harm the neck or cervical muscles. Now, return to the normal standing position with your hands by the side of your body. Repeat this exercise with the left hand on the back and the right hand clasping it. Rerun the exercise for at least 30-60 times with the timeline of clasped hands no less than 60-80 seconds.

(Refer to Illustration 6.10: **Gaumukh Aasan** गौमुखआसन *at Page No. 136)*

Chakra Swas Aasan चक्रस्वाँसआसन

An easy and basic exercise would be attempted in this subhead without undermining the outcome. Position yourself in sidh aasan सिद्धआसन or padma aasan पद्माआसन with bent elbows and, hands resting/fingers touching the shoulder. Following this posture, inhale deeply and hold the breath in lungs. To exhale, push the air out of the lungs whilst straightening your hands upwards. Repeat the exercise for at least 20-40 times, without resting in between. This exercise should stimulate your anahata chakra while delivering stimulations to mooldhara chakra too.

(Refer to Illustration 6.11: **Chakra Swas Aasan** चक्रस्वाँसआसन *at Page No. 137)*

Hand Formulations बंध

For organizing hand formulations बंध in this chakra, fingers associated with ether, air, fire and earth have to be assembled in such a way that the tip of thumb, middle finger and the ring finger touch each other and the index finger intersects this formation and touches the base of the thumb. With little finger fully stretched out, this बंध is called hridaya bandh. Sit in a relaxed pose and observe your breath before forming this बंध. Post its formation, if no change is observed in the breathing patterns, inspect if your back is bent and/or the fingers are converging at the appropriate point. Amend the variation and observe again.

(Refer to Illustration 6.12: **Hand Formulations** [Hridaya Mudra] *at Page No. 137)*

Focus-based Exercises ध्यानक्रिया

For an uninterrupted concentration on vishudhi chakra, you need to follow the breath, right from your nostrils to the bay point of the ribs and collar bone. Follow it both ways, while inhaling and exhaling. Now, try to alter your breathing without losing on the concentration of tracking your breath. Maintain the focus for a comfortable duration with an extended time period, which you deem fit for this chakra.

Mantras Recitation मंत्रउच्चारण

The following mantra needs to be recited for stimulating this chakra

HNHNHNHNNNNNNNNMMMMMHMHMHMHNMHNMH
NMHNM

Pertinently, the mantra needs to be recited whilst being breathless. In other words, you should fully exhale all the breath from within your chest before reciting this mantra. The duration of the recitation would depend upon the activation level of your anahata chakra. Due medical advice and permission should be sought before attempting this.

Naad Kriya ध्वनियोग

In order to accomplish this, place yourself in a silent room which is dark or dim lighted. Close your eyes and shift the focus to your throat. You have the option to swallow your saliva for a smooth experience. Maintain the focus on your throat and try to engage your hearing with the chakra. Take notice of the flow of blood in your throat and slowly you would be able to sense the flow of energy, both inwards and outwards. While upholding the focus and with regular and sincere practice, one should be able to hear the sounds, as produced by this chakra. Initially, they may sound faint, but with enhanced concentration, the notes of music would appear distinct.

Yantra Sadhna यंत्रसाधना

This yantra of root chakra is formed by configuring the body (using hands/arms, legs) in such a way that when you breathe, the stimulations caused by the usual posture of the body occur in the root chakra. For root chakra, twist your legs in a manner that they entangle/grope each other while standing. Repeat the same for arms too, while ensuring that at the point where groping of arms ends, the palms face each other.

Hold onto this position while maintaining a normal breath. Now, gently entangle your arms and legs, and relax by engaging in routine stretching exercises. You can repeat the process again while making sure that the holding period of this formulation should be at least 20 minutes (inclusive of the repetitions), initially. Down the line, one may choose to increase it as, per the strength and endurance.

Tantra Sadhna तंत्रसाधना

This facet of the chakra meditation is beyond the ambit of this book.

Illustrative Representation of Aasana's

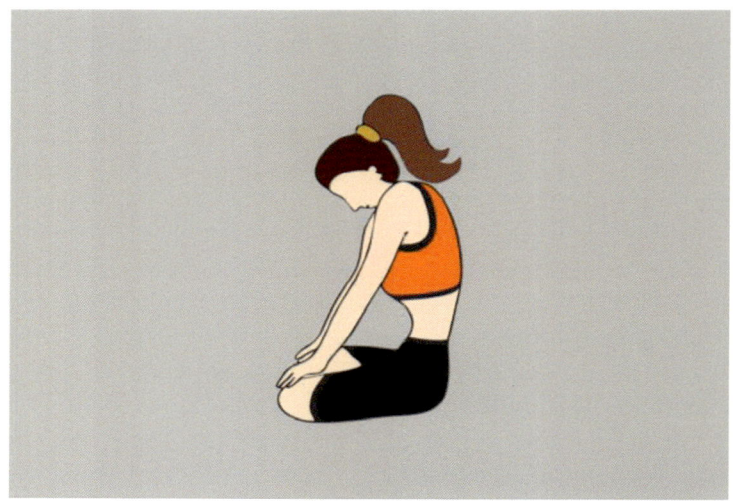

Illustration 6.1: Jallandhar Bandh Yog जालंधरबंधयोग

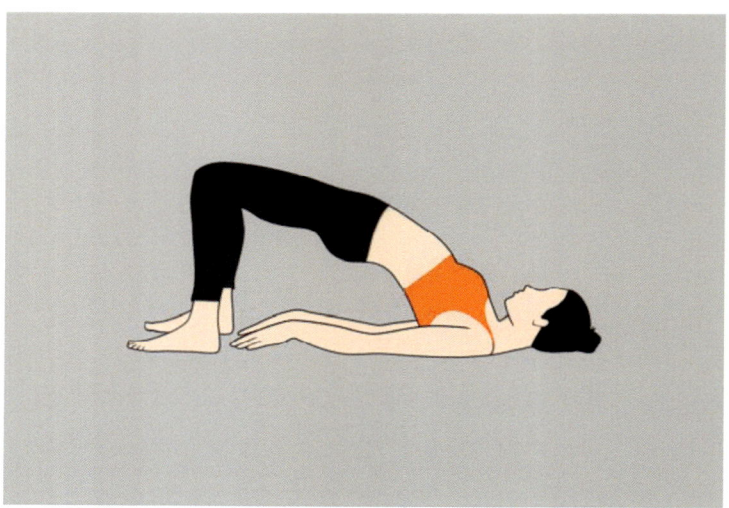

Illustration 6.2: Setu Bandh Sarvang Aasan सेतुबंधसर्वांगआसन

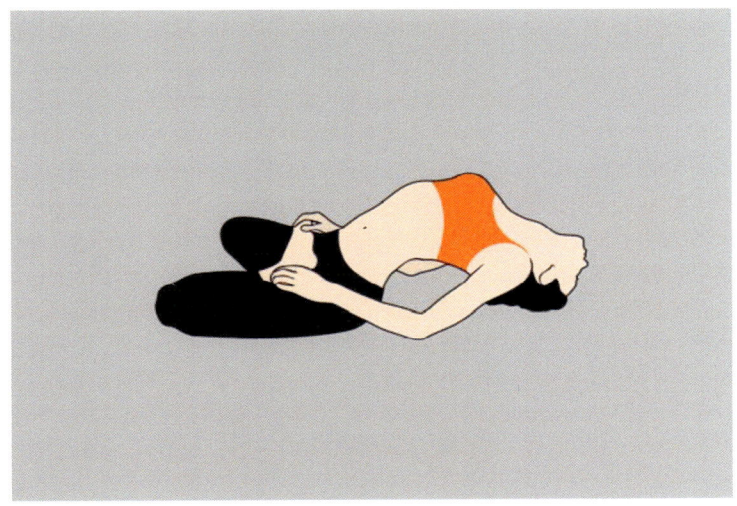

Illustration 6.3: Mtsaya Aasan मत्स्यआसन

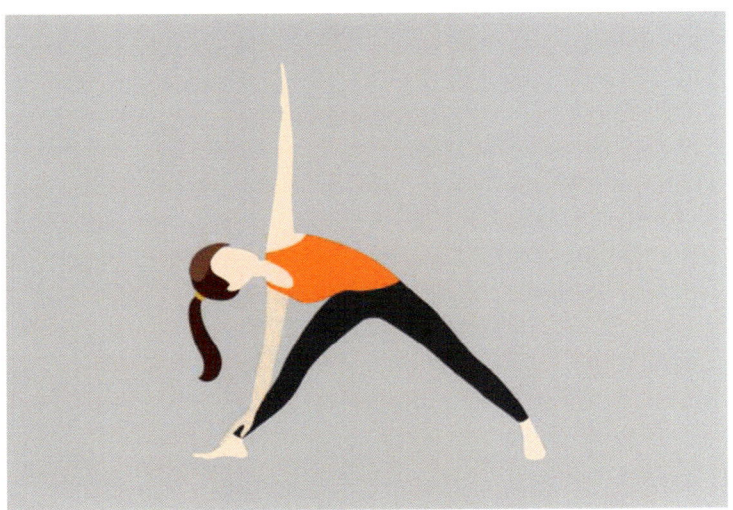

Illustration 6.4: Trikon Aasan त्रिकोणआसन

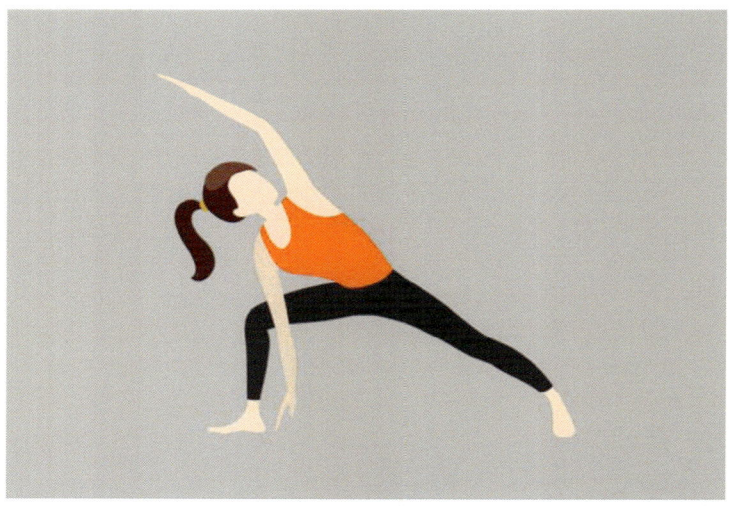

Illustration 6.5: Parivrata Prasarvkon Aasan परिवृत्त पर्सर्वकोणआसन

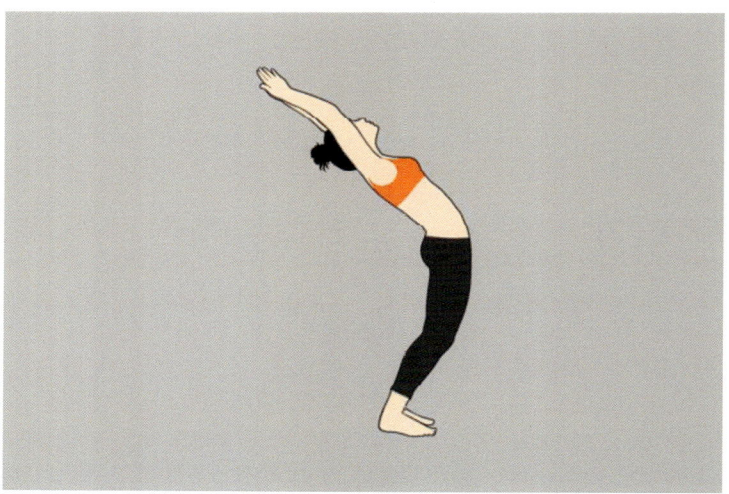

Illustration 6.6: Ardh Chandra Aasan अर्धचंद्रआसन

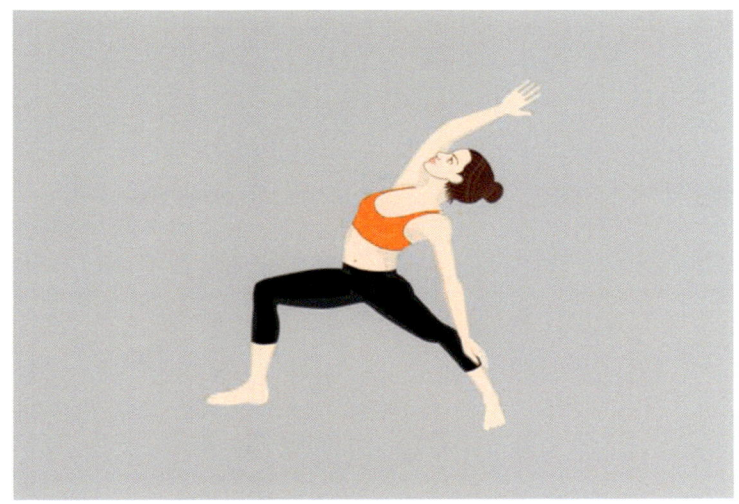

Illustration 6.7: Viprit Virbhadar Aasan विप्रीतवीरभद्रआसन

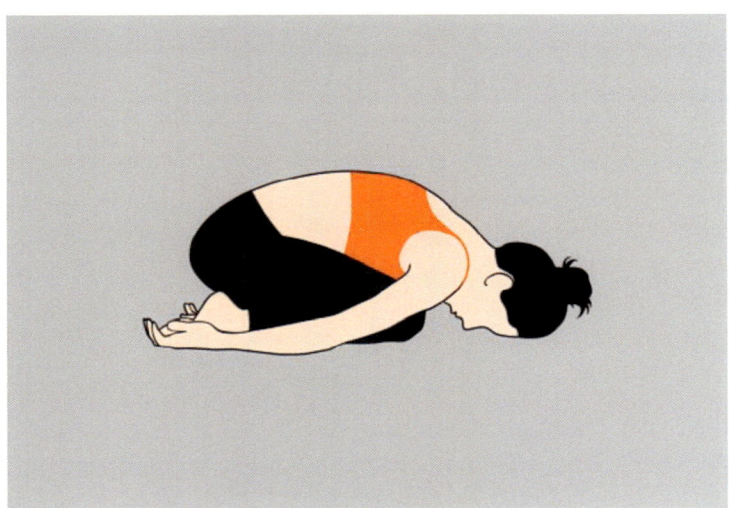

Illustration 6.8: Yog Mudra योगमुद्रा

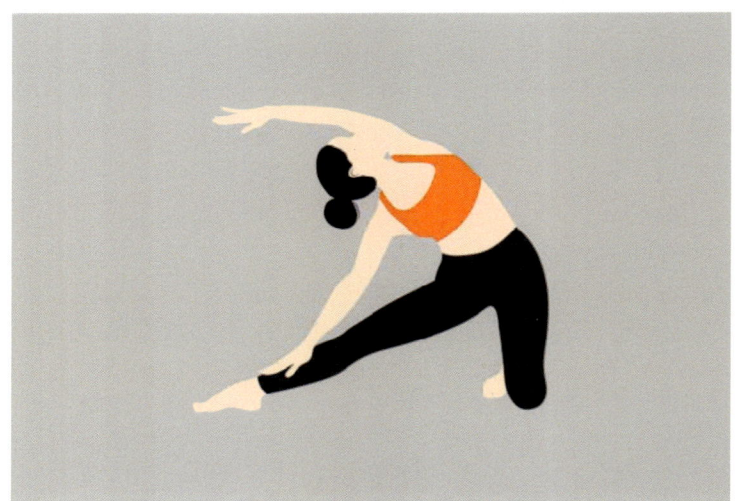

Illustration 6.9: Parig Aasan प्रिगआसन

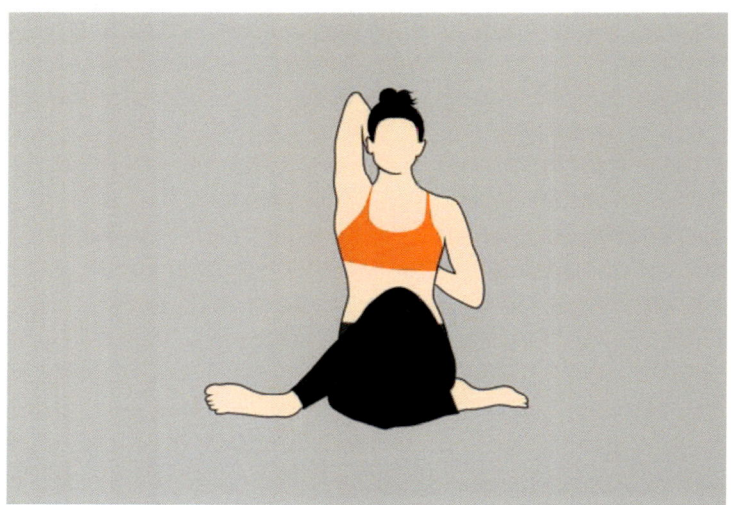

Illustration 6.10: Gaumukh Aasan गौमुखआसन

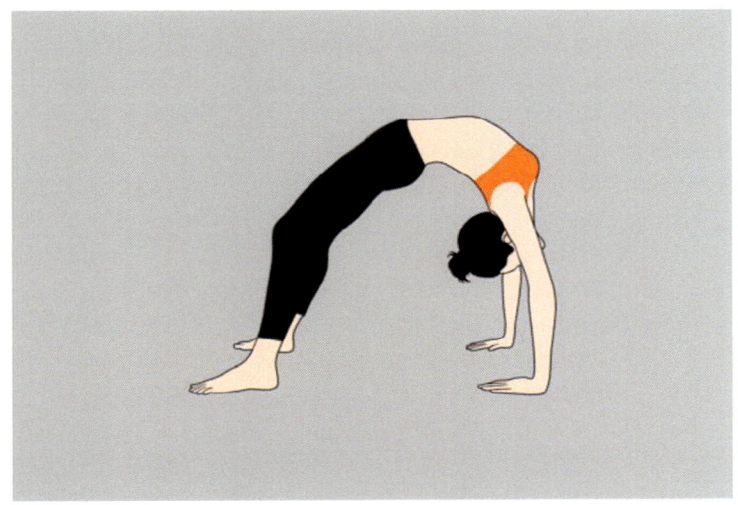

Illustration 6.11: Chakra Swas Aasan चक्रस्वाँसआसन

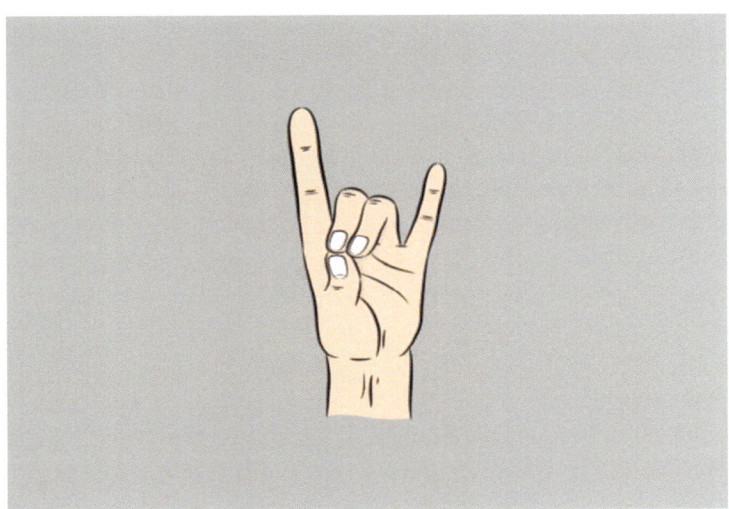

Illustration 6.12: Hand Formulations [Hridaya Mudra]

7
Agya Chakra: Space and Ether

वज्रख्याविंयाकतअदेसेवलसतीसातम: कर्णिक्यमध्यस्थानमकोणम:
तत्तरैपूर्खमतदीदिव्याविलस्त: कोमलमकामरूपमकंदर्पोंनाम:
वायूरनिवस्तीसतात्म: तस्यामध्येसामंत: जीवोबंधुजीवाप्रक्रमभिहासं:
कोटिसूर्याप्रकाश:!

The mouth of the nadi is called vajra and in the pericarp, exists a beautiful, luminous and soft, constantly shining lightening-like triangle karmarupa, known as Traipura. The presence of vayu called kandarpa is omnipresent, which is of a deeper red colour like the bandhujiva flower, and is the Lord of Beings and resplendent like ten million suns.

The tri-conjunction of mooldhara chakra in the pericarp is aptly portrayed. The triangle, according to visvanatha and gautamiya tantra is iccha-jnana-kriyatmaka (the powers of will, knowledge, and action). The triangle is the charming sakti pitha, above dhara-bija. The three lines are VAmA, JyestA and Raudri.

This chakra is placed at glabella (space between the eyebrows). It is at this place on the forehead, one feels the sensations the time this chakra is activated. In Sanskrit language, this chakra is called the agya chakra आज्ञाचक्र, which in the English language, would translate to, the one which "commands". At this point of confluence, the scope, provisions and possibilities of matter are off, and the life energies step into a "new domain", which is beyond shapes and figures. In the Vedic system, the beej mantras for this chakra are recited in a manner encompassing exclusive inhaling followed by complete exhaling. It can also be implied in the sense of irrelevance of air reaching the organs or while being there. Simply putting, it is relevant only for this chakra, when enroute. To elucidate, there is no start or end point, as far as the activation of this chakra is concerned, since element earth is not a contributory factor in this chakra.

As described in yog vashisht, this chakra has two petals, both of which are prominent as well as dominant. This chakra is what we recognize as the "pituitary gland"—the master gland of the body. If observed diligently, the stimulations generated by the recitation of the beej mantras of this chakra, create ripples and pulses, demonstrating a distinctive effect on pituitary gland. When a person is able to master concentration and focus, there is an enhanced realization about the effects being communicated to this gland.

The inward and outward flow of energy from this chakra can be perceived in the form of a shapeless structure (according to my experience). To confer it a name, "ellipsoid" would be a suitable option, as it is almost impossible to define it within the periphery of a definite shape. Example of the never ending flame of a candle, determined by the length of the wick, would be a handy correlation to the notion, greater the concentration, greater would be the flow of energy in this chakra.

The ethos of stimulating and activating this chakra lies in the ability to focus. Lack of focus would render scant possibilities of sensing this chakra. All three major nerves viz. ida, pingla and sushumna ईड़ा, पिंगला और सुषुम्ना, while embarking on their upward journey from the mooldhara chakra मूलधाराचक्र, convene at this chakra.

Ida and pingla ईड़ा और पिंगला take the outward route from here, hosting themselves at the back of the ears, in the chakras. From here onwards, sushumna सुषुम्ना starts its journey upwards, possessing the combined energies of both ida and pingla ईड़ा और पिंगला nerves.

इडाभागीरथीगंगापिंगलायमुनानदीतयोर्मध्यर्गतानाडीसुषुम्नासरस्वती

The above verse can be inferred as follows. Ida ईड़ा and pingla पिंगला are like rivers Ganga and Yamuna. Sushumna सुषुम्ना is like river Saraswati सरस्वती, flowing in the middle of the two. It is here, in agya chakra आज्ञाचक्र, that the confluence संगम of energy happens. This is the point from where one starts the journey, beyond the body. At this juncture, you are beyond the body to realise that you are not just a body. This confluence point is the turf where one gets blessed by Lord Shiva. Shiv, which is a Sanskrit word, can be translated as, "the one which isn't but without whom there can be nothing". As mentioned above, in this chakra, there is no shape or figure, but without it, there is no possibility of having any shape or size.

The time you would be able to activate this chakra, the same would have a trickling effect on your societal association, in addition to providing you a scope for the spiritual world. There are six major virtues in terms of societal connection, which are experienced, post the activation of this chakra. These are:
1. Intellect
2. Power to manifest, by just having its thought
3. Fearlessness
4. The one who can host anything
5. Recoiling of virtue
6. Power to guide

There would be no engagement of the sensory system for activation of this chakra. One won't visualize or see any kind of light or lights and nor would you be detecting any sound. There would be nothing in this chakra, which you shall be able to express in words. Simply stating, since all that you have experienced is beyond the sensory body, therefore, if you have witnessed things which you are in a position to communicate or share with others, you are definitely not executing the same in a correct manner. Whatever you have accomplished, is just a hallucination.

In any case, if one is focusing on the agya chakra and the following virtues are visible and prominent, one can be confident of treading the established path.

1) Your presence is solicited and welcomed.
2) You have a greater perception of having the sense of events before their occurrence, and have the ability to change the course and hence the result of those events.
3) You do not carry any kind of emotions or passion, even if you are condoned or condemned.
4) You speak less; your vocal articulation is only to promulgate truth and clarify any myths.
5) Although you involved in the act, yet untouched by its outcome.
6) You do not regard anyone as a physical entity but rather your association is based upon the energies inherent in another person.
7) You are wealthy and satisfied.
8) You normally don't fall sick, and your diet is determined by hunger and not by the timing.

It is the confluence of these three nerves viz. ida, pingla and sushumna ईड़ा, पिंगला और सुषुम्ना in the designated space, that the energy develops newer formulations and is all together different. There is no heat or coldness and in addition, there is no recognition of the sensory system. Presumably, there can be no definition of this unnoticeable and unrecognisable "energy", rejuvenated by high voltages. Focus on these points of conductivity, in a specific location, is the ethos of this chakra.

The synapse between the two hemispheres of the brain is the point where the two petals of this chakra meet each other. It is here, that the energy goes beyond the societal and emotional sense and realises higher energies. Post this realization, i.e. following the activation of agya chakra, a person in the real sense, starts understanding the spiritual world and its intricacies.

Consciousness about yourself, till now, has been your association with the body and its senses and how and what the societal norms have been. In this chakra, you go beyond all these. Embodied in this chakra, is the ability to realise that consciousness integrates a lot more than just the ones mentioned above. There would be consciousness about the "energy body", which has been there all this while, but you have been ignorant about it. This subtle energy is too eager to meet its Shiva, but the path isn't clear and there is nothing to support its movement. Our perceptions and convictions about the emotional life has been a contributory factor in blocking its path and, hence the abode. The idea of perceptions is obvious and overcoming them extends a possibility to sight a vision, thereby facilitating the capability to enter into agya chakra.

Existence of perceptions and convictions would hinder entry into this space, as there is nothing in this chakra which can have a "shape", and convictions and perceptions are nothing more or less than psychological shapes of your own thoughts and concepts. Pineal gland is a part of the brain, which gets stimulated during the process of activating this chakra. This happens parallel to the creation of stimulations in the pituitary gland, followed by greater secretion of positive and healthy hormones like serotonin.

During the period when a person is awake, sense is greatly driven by seeing or vision. While employing sight, things that one witnesses, drives the emotions. Interestingly, it is this sight that generates the corresponding emotions. As to what you perceive of that sight—liking or disliking—ultimately generates those emotions. However, this undergoes a transformation the time agya chakra is activated. It is the inner vision which eventually takes over, as the release of DMT neurotransmitter happens, post stimulations in the pineal gland. But, these inner visions are not something you would be seeing with your open eyes. As observed in a number of cases, the person sees himself as another person (what is normally referred as out of the body experience).

Yog will guide you in a direction towards a deeper and inner self and a newer outer world, with sight and light having an all together different meaning. This shift, devoid of perceptions and convictions, is what will happen, post activation of the agya chakra. Many a school of thoughts advocate the concept of a guided activation (called hallucination in psychology). Under its purview, a pupil/client is made to drive and direct the emotions on a prescribed path, stemming the sensations in the glabella area which further trickle down into the pineal gland. This kind of activation or speculated activation may effectuate a sense of having the agya chakra activated but whether it is really activated or not, could be anyone's guess. As a part of my teaching, I would facilitate this path for you. Difficult as it may seem, my prerogative is to help you achieve this course of action.

There are a few pertinent physical yog postures, considered suitable in activating this chakra. However, as mentioned in vishudhi chakra also, there is very little that a physical body can do for the activation of these two chakras (as there is nothing which a physical body can do for the activation of the sahastrdhara chakra).

Breathing स्वाँस

For stimulating this chakra, you need to focus on the movements occurring in your midline and spine area when you are breathing. Simply putting, while inhaling and exhaling, you need to monitor the observations in these areas. The greater the observation better would be the scope to stimulate the chakra and its resultant activation. If one is diligently noticing the breath, there would be a realization, of change in its temperature when confined to the nostrils and the time it is gone past the throat area and reaches lungs. This process can be adopted to master the observational qualities, following which one is able to recognise the variations occurring in the spine clearly. Variations would be noticeable in ripple/tingling and their intensity and concentration can also be ascertained;

as these changes vary from being significant to just minute. Undoubtedly, their presence is indisputable, as while inhaling, you will observe a tendency among them to move towards the direction from where the breath is being sucked in. Ultimately, this reverses and they start moving in the opposite direction when you exhale. This translates into a change in position which it has been holding till now, and you would be pleasantly surprised to register their presence, hitherto unrecognised and unrealised by you.

Physical Yog योग

There are a few movements which I normally ask the clients to perform. Basically, these are rapid eye movements from the right to the left and from top to the bottom before proceeding towards attempting physical postures of the body. The objective behind these eye movements is to relax the eyes, glabella and the forehead area in addition to taking away the thoughts from the brain.

Kapalbhatti कपालभाटी

For performing this aasan, you can choose to be either in sidh aasan सिद्धआसन or padma aasan पद्माआसन. Increase the breathing rate, which means you have to inhale and exhale as fast you can. However, in both the cases, the muscles in your abdominal area should either contract or stretch. Doing this exercise without engagement of the abdominal muscle would be a waste of time and energy with no fruitful results. This exercise when done in a correct manner, helps in the release of toxins from body and also aids in relieving body and mind of stress.

(Refer to Illustration 7.1: **Kapalbhatti** कपालभाटी *at Page No. 151)*

Lom Vilom लोमविलोम

For this aasan also, you can choose to sit in either sidh aasan सिद्धआसन or padma aasan पद्माआसन. Engage your thumb to press your right nostril and inhale from the left nostril. Here onwards, while exhaling, use your ring and little finger to press the left nostril and breathe out from your right nostril. Repeat this exercise as many times as you can while maintaining the stretching and contraction stance of your abdominal muscles.

(Refer to Illustration 7.2: **Lom Vilom** लोमविलोम *at Page No. 151)*

Virbhadhra Aasan वीरभद्रआसन

This aasan derives its name from a form of Lord Shiva, namely, Virbhadra. In this form, Lord Shiva is in an angry mood. For performing this aasan, stand straight with an erect back and then move your right leg forward and bend its knee. While holding this position, stretch your head with spread fingers of your hand over your head as if one is trying to catch something. Breathe fast and heavy while maintaining this pose. Continue the breathing as long as you can comfortably and then return to the standing position. Now, relax and repeat the exercise with left leg forward. Do ensure that the time period for both the legs remains the same and uniform number of breaths are inhaled and exhaled with either of leg stretched forward.

(Refer to Illustration 7.3: **Virbhadhra Aasan** वीरभद्रआसन *at Page No. 152)*

Viprit Virbhadhra Aasan विप्रीतवीरभद्रआसन

For performing this aasan, you need to be standing straight with an erect back. Now, from this position, stretch your legs sideways till you are comfortable holding on to that position. Now, turn your torso towards the right leg and raise your right hand above your head while keeping your left hand on the thigh or knee of the straight and stretched left leg and bend the right knee. Let your head follow your hand making and bend a little backwards as if you are watching the fingers of your right hand. Hold on to this position while maintaining a heavy and hard breathing. Hold as long as you are comfortable and then return to the position of stretched legs while keeping the torso straight. Relax before performing this exercise on the other side. This aasan has proven beneficial in providing strength to the legs, abdominal area and shoulders in addition to extending flexibility.

(Refer to Illustration 7.4: **Viprit Virbhadhra Aasan** विप्रीतवीरभद्रआसन *at Page No. 152)*

Setu Bandha Sarvangaasan सेतुबंधसर्वांगआसन

In this aasan आसन, you need to lie down on your back, with legs stretched forward. Now, bend your knees and lift your pelvis while keeping your shoulders and head on the ground. Hold onto this position and bring your arms in the space created by lifting up of your lower torso and let the hands clip together. Hold this position for as long as possible, and when you choose to return, first untangle the hands and move your arms to the side of the body and gently let your body touch the ground. As your torso has touched the ground slowly, stretch your legs forward and relax before repeating the exercise.

(Refer to Illustration 7.5: **Setu Bandha Sarvangaasan** सेतुबंधसर्वांगआसन *at Page No. 153)*

Mtsaya Aasan मत्स्यआसन

To carry out this aasan, lie down on your back with your hands comfortably resting around the waist area. Now, try and bend your head inwards so that your chest and shoulders are slightly lifted from the floor while keeping your hands on the ground. Try to accommodate the entire load of chest and shoulders on your neck area without any assistance from arms. Maintain this position for as long as you can, without inviting any strain on the neck, back, and cervical area. It is essential not to hold the stretched position while feeling breathless, ensuring that breathing remains normal.

(Refer to Illustration 7.6: **Mtsaya Aasan** मत्स्यआसन *at Page No. 153)*

Trikon Aasan त्रिकोणआसन

For performing this aasan, you need to stand straight with an erect back. Now, stretch your legs sideways to the position as you are comfortable holding it there and able to balance yourself. While in this position, move your right arm to the back of your right leg in a manner that you are able to hold the heel of your right leg and move your left arm over your head and place your head in a position as if you are following your left arm and are able to see the fingers of your left hand. Hang on to this position while holding the breath inside you. Hold this position for as long as you can before returning to the standing position with your legs stretched sideways. Relax your body and try to breathe normally, before repeating this exercise on the other side. This aasan helps in improving digestion and provides great relief from stiff legs and hips and has also been found beneficial in easing sciatica pain.

(Refer to Illustration 7.7: **Trikon Aasan** त्रिकोणआसन *at Page No. 154)*

Phalaasan पलआसन

For performing this aasan, lie down on your belly and lift yourself with bended elbows in an effort to form a plank. Try and keep your entire body in a straight line and keep your head in a forward looking position while keeping your breath normal. Maintain this position as per your comfort levels without feeling breathlessness. This aasana increases the strength of abdominal muscles in addition to strengthening legs, chest and shoulders.

(Refer to Illustration 7.8: **Phalaasan** पलआसन *at Page No. 154)*

Vashishth Aasan वशिष्ठआसन

For performing this aasan, you need to lie on your high side. Now, lift your body sideways using the right hand. Lift your body till the time the right hand becomes fully stretched and keep your feet joined, with one placed over the other.

(Refer to Illustration 7.9: **Vashishth Aasan** वशिष्ठआसन *at Page No. 155)*

Salbhas Aasan सलभसआसन

For performing this aasan, you need to lie down on your belly with arms around the waist area. From this position, lift your head, chest and legs while keeping your arms in the air. Hold on to this position for a while and try sustaining your breath as long as you can comfortably. Now, return to the first position of lying down on your belly. Relax for a while before repeating the exercise.

(Refer to Illustration 7.10: **Salbhas Aasan** सलभसआसन *at Page No. 155)*

Supta Padangusthasan सुप्तपदंगुस्तआसन

In this aasan आसन, the inner muscles of the legs and the bridge joining the legs are stimulated, which helps in activating the root chakra.

Spread your arms completely at shoulder height and then lift your leg and try and touch the hand of that side while rotating your head in the opposite direction. Repeat the same exercise on other side also, whilst ensuring that there is no stress on the back and there is a feeling of stimulations on the "bridge" of the legs.

(Refer to Illustration 7.11: **Supta Padangusthasan** सुप्तपदंगुस्तआसन *at Page No. 156)*

Ustr Aasan उत्त्रआसन

For performing this aasan, sit on the bent knees whilst keeping your spine erect and shoulders comfortably spread and the chest area protruding out. Now place your hands on the waist, and push the chest further in front while bending your spine backwards. The degree of bending the spine is entirely dependent on your flexibility levels. Further, touch the heels of the feet with your hands and maintain this position for a significant period. Under no circumstances, try and overdo, as it may prove detrimental for the back.

(Refer to Illustration 7.12: **Ustr Aasan** उत्त्रआसन *at Page No. 156)*

Bhujang Aasan भुजंगआसन

For performing this aasan, lie down on your belly and bring your folded arms close to your chest and using the strength of your arms with the support of spine muscles, lift your upper torso from the ground while keeping your pelvis and lower torso on the ground. Now, lift your body and stretch backwards while keeping the maximum weight on the arms, which would be almost straight by now. Remain in this position as per your comforting levels and slowly return to the position of lying on your belly.

*(Refer to Illustration 7.13: **Bhujang Aasan** भुजंगआसन at Page No. 157)*

Apanaasan अपानआसन

As you are aware, the root chakra is at the tip of the spine. This aasan आसन, helps in stimulating the tip and the corresponding muscles of the area. Lie down on your back with your legs extended forward, and slowly bend your knees one by one or at one go, depending on the existing strength of the pelvis area (at no point of time, stretch yourself beyond your comfortable limits) and move these bent knees towards the chest area.

You will experience the lifting of the tip and of the spine too. It is okay if it rises above the ground but do try to keep it to the ground while moving your bent knees towards the chest. When your knees have come close to the chest, grope them with your arms and hold them while keeping your breathing normal.

Release the position and gently place your feet on the ground in forward extended position and relax and keep your head and rest of the body on the floor. Now, slightly lift your legs, hold them and then release. At this point, you should be feeling some sensation in the tip of the spine. In case you are not that observant, you can feel the change in the muscles surrounding the spine.

*(Refer to Illustration 7.14: **Apanaasan** अपानआसन at Page No. 157)*

Hand Formulations बंध

Yoni mudra योनिमुद्रा is the बंध for this aasan. For forming this mudra, join the tips of your index fingers and those of your thumbs in a position that they are repulsing each other and placed at the opposite ends. Form this mudra and observe the changes in breathing and the movement of energy within.

(Refer to Illustration 7.15: **Hand Formulations** [Yoni Mudra] *at Page No. 158)*

Focus-based Exercises ध्यानक्रिया

This is a major key for stimulating and activating this chakra. The focus should be maintained above the eyes around the forehead area. At no point, you should let the focus shift to any other place in your system, or try hallucinating. Imagine things and aim to generate a "feel good" rather than "being good" element.

Mantras Recitation मंत्रउच्चारण

The mantra for this chakra should be recited in the following manner to obtain the best results

HAOMSHAOMHMHMHMHAINHAINHAIN

Before reciting this mantra, keep the chest area without breath, which means exhale out fully.

Illustrative Representation of Aasana's

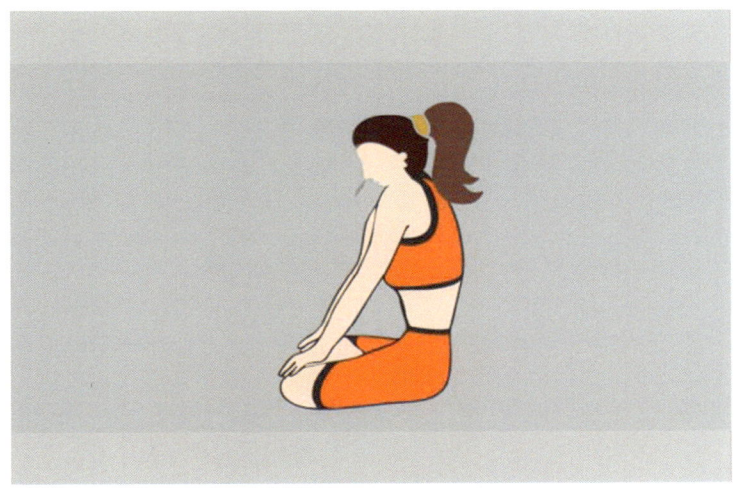

Illustration 7.1: Kapalbhatti कपालभाटी

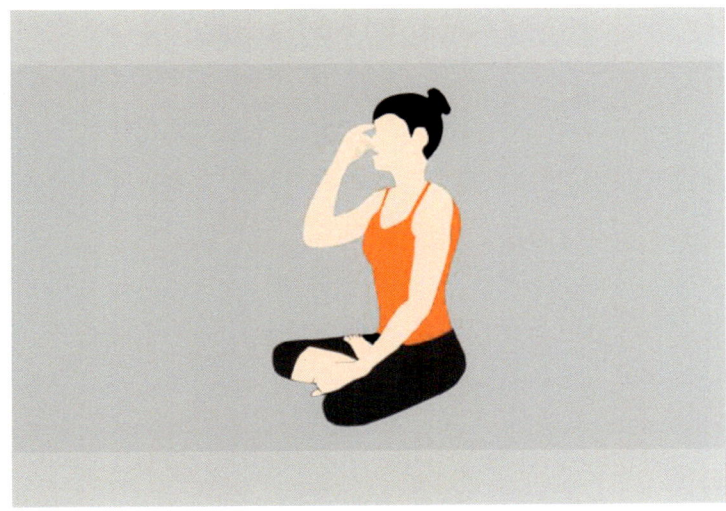

Illustration 7.2: Lom Vilom लोमविलोम

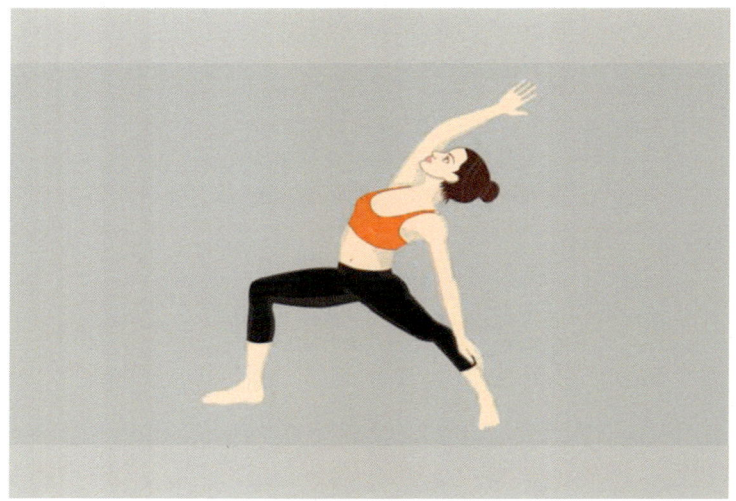

Illustration 7.3: Virbhadhra Aasan वीरभद्रआसन

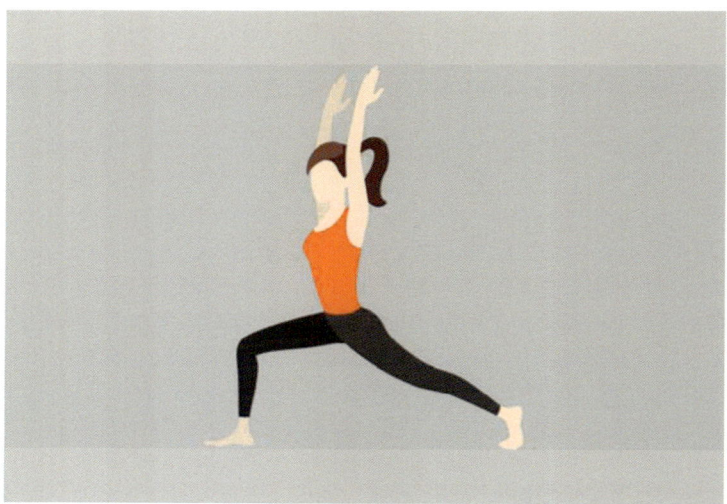

Illustration 7.4: Viprit Virbhadhra Aasan विप्रीतवीरभद्रआसन

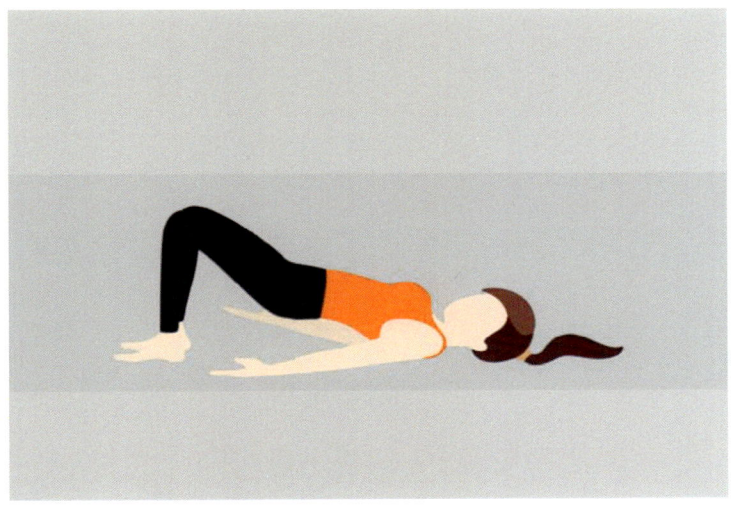

Illustration 7.5: Setu Bandha Sarvangaasan सेतुबंधसर्वांगआसन

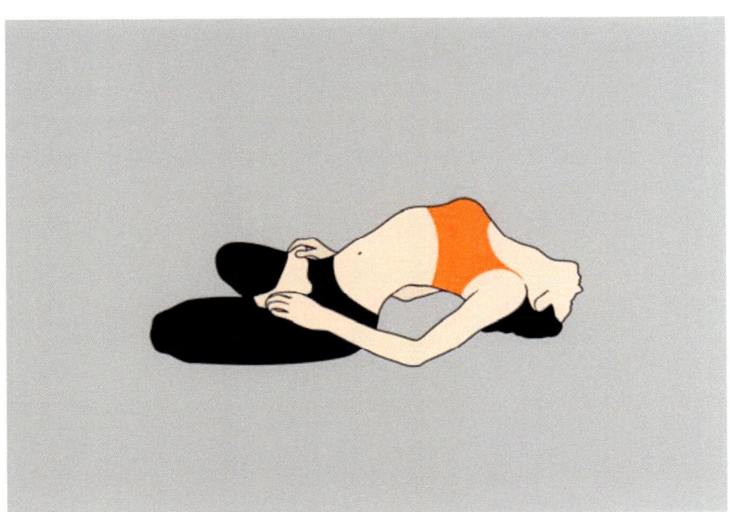

Illustration 7.6: Mtsaya Aasan मत्स्यआसन

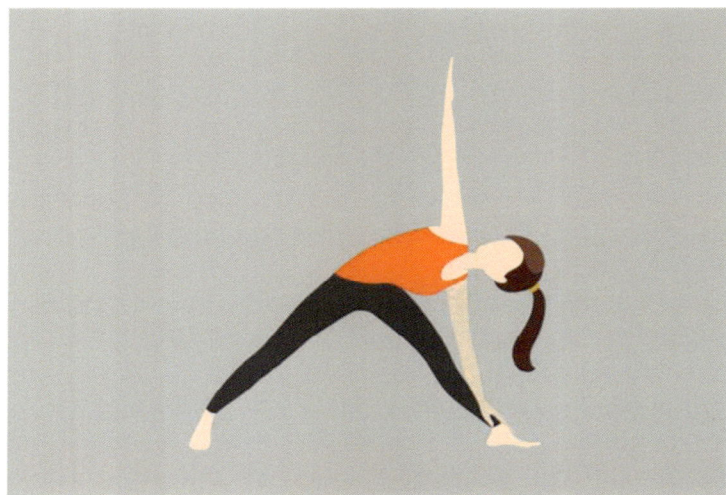

Illustration 7.7: Trikon Aasan त्रिकोणआसन

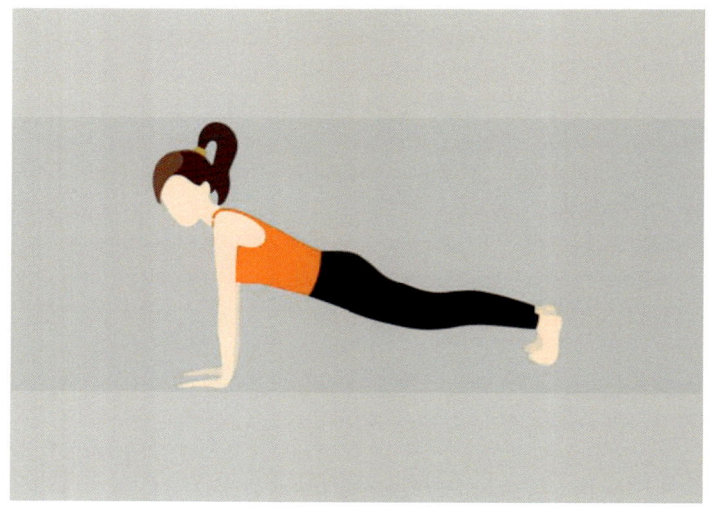

Illustration 7.8: Phalaasan पलआसन

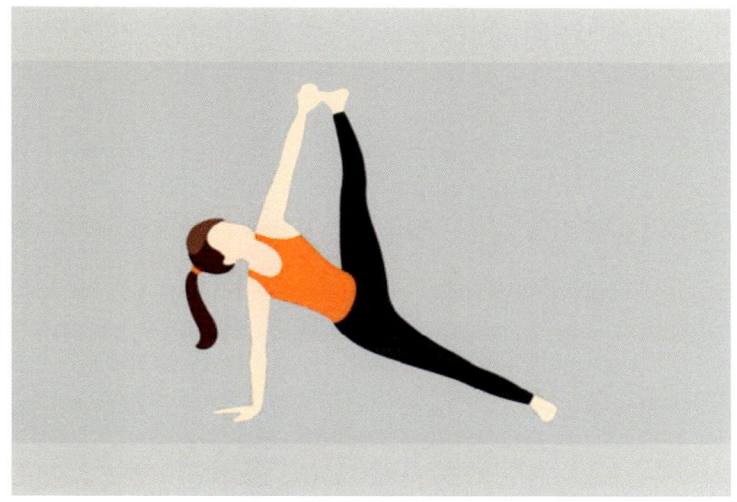

Illustration 7.9: Vashishth Aasan वशिष्ठआसन

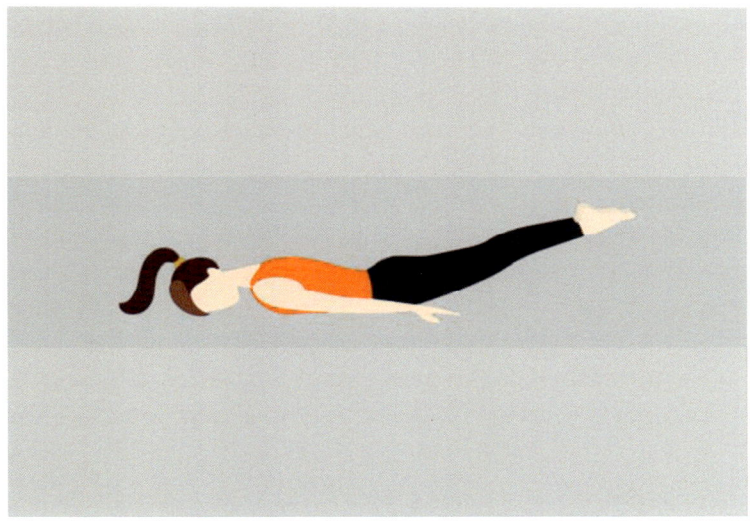

Illustration 7.10: Salbhas Aasan सलभसआसन

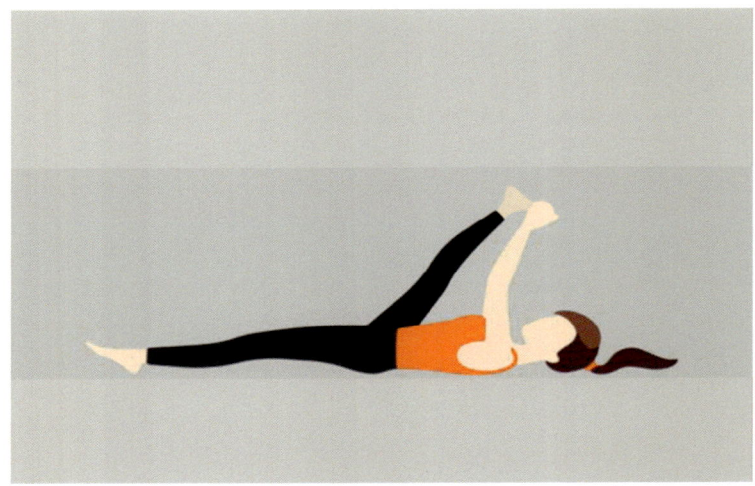

Illustration 7.11: Supta Padangusthasan सुप्तपदंगुस्तआसन

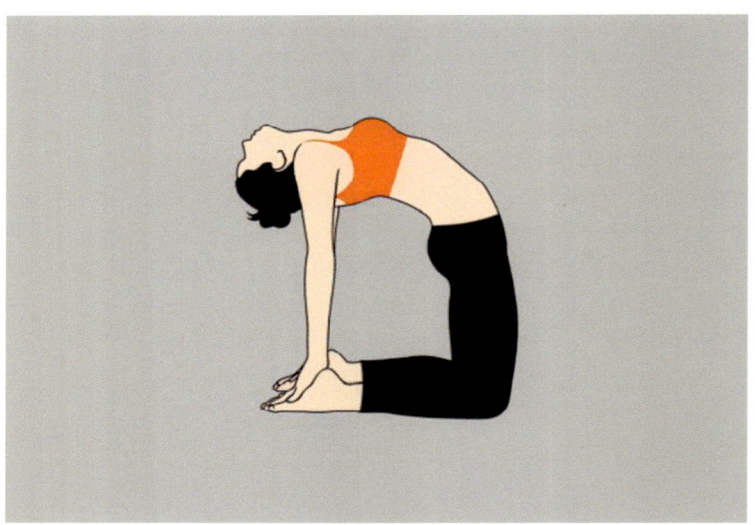

Illustration 7.12: Ustr Aasan उस्त्रआसन

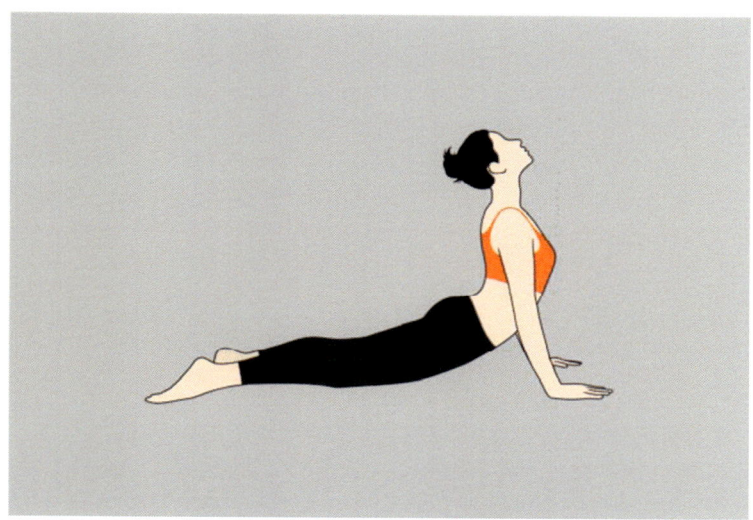

Illustration 7.13: Bhujang Aasan भुजंगआसन

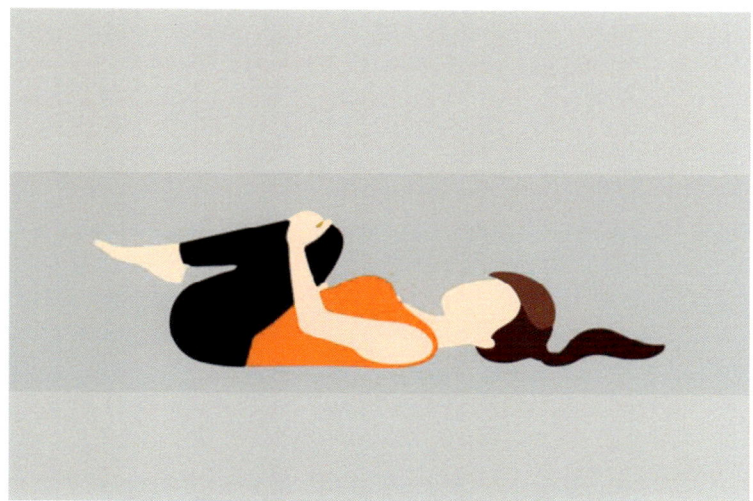

Illustration 7.14: Apanaasan अपानआसन

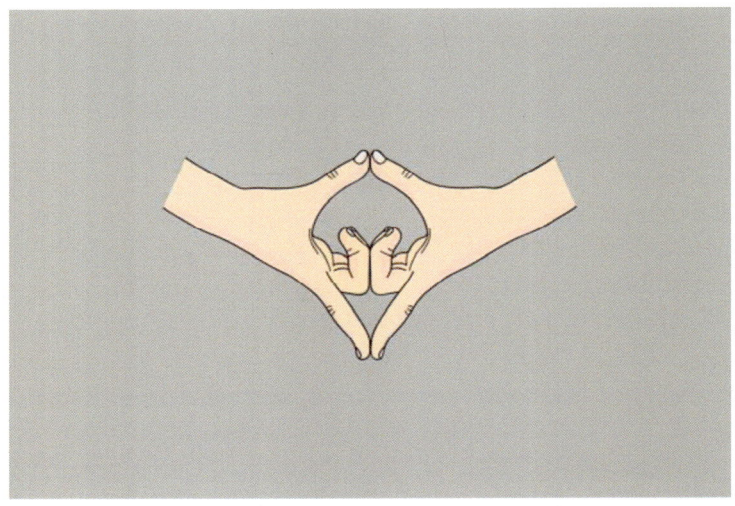

Illustration 7.15: Hand Formulations [Yoni Mudra)

8

The Principles for Kundalini Awakening

While embarking on the course of kundalini awakening, the place for carrying out the proceedings assumes significance. Any location in the midst of nature, preferably, a park where there is silence, or a water body, viz. a pond or a flowing river, or in the country side, would be ideal choices. Choice of a venue is essential and, instrumental in enhancing the intensity of the elements inside the body by the surrounding ambience, which should provide a sense of comfort, peace and solace by its very sight. One has to be comfortable and no emotions should be attached with the place upon completion of the regime at you end. The comfort level of the place should be reflected in your inclination to frequent the place, irrespective of the regimen, just to be in harmony with nature.

The connotation of a place in simple terms would mean, a place which has the provisions of taking you away from your thoughts; a place which is not only visited by people who want to practice yog or meditation, rather the very inherent nature of that place attracts people towards it; a place where birds are chirping and flora and fauna is in abundance.

The place where you wish to performing yog and meditation, should inculcate a sense of belongingness. The perception should be distinct from what you experience in a man-made brick and mortar structure. It is important to establish connect between yourself and the place to feel the wholeness. Being at such a place physically would transpire a sense of jubilation and revival, and/or even the thought of heading to that place would generate a feeling of joy.

Certain intrinsic characteristics of the natural surroundings should also be evident. The trees should be fruit bearing and not thorny, as fruit bearing trees have the possibility to attract a diverse number of birds, resonating an active ecosystem. The sizeable mass of the trees having deep roots would also be conducive in transmitting the association of element earth with an evolving life, i.e. you. In addition, these deep roots are a reflection of how element water can be felt even when it is not visible. Since, the water underground, is not visible to the naked eye, so is the case with element air which is pristine in its actuality, as while flowing through the dense trees, it carries along with it, the richness of element water (in the form of water vapours and/or droplets).

Nature lovers would connect with this kind of ambience intrinsically, to enjoy its glory and drawing a parallel with the sub-stratosphere, supportive enough to assist in your endeavour towards activating the kundalini. Banking on the logic too, what is within you and around you being all natural, without any fabrication of things, it would augur well for an unhindered journey so desired. As described and suggested above, the location should preferably be rich in fruit bearing trees with an abundance of flora and fauna. This would also ensure a soothing weather. The current of air and the breath of wind, brushing past your face and body during its flow, will help you to relax and be away from any kind of adamantine traits or virtues/concepts. You should be able to envisage that the sense of change is "inevitable" and you are welcoming it to happen. Prevailing thoughts and emotions should last during the entire duration of stay at that place. The smile on your face should not be an act which you have to think about. The pristine and solace providing place should in itself be enough for that smile to remain on your face at all the times.

One may have been blessed with lots of fortunes and riches, but they can be truly cherished when the energy within, is in your favour. A person can buy delicious food and delicacies, but not the hunger and the capacity to eat and digest the same. Likewise, all individuals do possess kundalini power, but to activate itself or to remain in a dormant state, the decision lies solely with the power itself. It is only subsequently that a person develops the fervour to deliberate and ponder over this "hidden science". While glancing over this book and as a reader, you have been fortunate enough to tread this path.

The time kundalini moves upwards from the mooldhara, which is also known as "mukt triveni" मुक्तत्रिवेणी, and starts moving from each chakra, one witnesses varying experiences. As is discernible, in swadisthana chakra, the ability to pre-sense the things is noticeable and when it moves upwards to manipura chakra, the aura of a person changes. The person is invited and welcomed and his presence is cherished by people around. Further, when it moves to anahata chakra, an augmentation in love and compassion is visible in a person, marked by empathy and compassion for others. When kundalini moves to vishudhi chakra, also called as "yukt triveni" युक्तत्रिवेणी, an introduction to cosmic phonemes happens. Experiences in agay and sahastrdhara cannot be explained or shared as they are beyond the scope of senses and unjustified to be narrated in words. Another facet of kundalini awakening can also be correlated to short-term health related issues like blood pressure, insomnia, and low pulse rate. However, this should not be a matter of concern as when the physical body gains strength to host the awakened kundalini's power, these ailments would recede.

Our spinal cord is made up of 33 types of bones, and kundalini moves through all these 33 types and encompasses a variable form of energy in each of them. That is the reason, in Hinduism, 33 types of Gods have been mentioned. All these 33 types of bones in the spinal cord are hollow from within and are interlinked. The last segment of the spinal cord is termed as tail bone and the area around the tail bone is identical to a bud. It is this area, where kundalini, the "serpentine power", sleeps and is hosted, but in a dormant state. To state a comparable representation, one may have all the beautiful chandeliers and impressive electric fixtures, but no power to light them up. Going by this example, it is the kundalini, which has the power to lighten up the prospects of your fortunes turning into realities. This is the time when your aspirations don't just remain your wishes but get manifested into actualities. It won't be a contradiction to remark that poor aren't poor because of poverty or lack of funds, rather it is due to the unrealised "power" within. This connotation should not be interpreted as, that wealthy people have awakened their kundalini, but it is the levels of activated chakras that they have been born with, which have effectuated their current standing. You too have those provisions and need a head start to activate the kundalini power within and be a witness to your progression.

There are 11 major nerves, present in the body. Among these, the prominent ones are, ida, pingla and sushumna (host to the vajrani वज्रानी nerve). This nerve originates from the shishan area and culminates at agya chakra. The two main nerves, viz. ida and pingla, are in a position in which they can grope the spinal cord and move in all the 114 chakras. On the other hand, sushumna is a nerve which moves from within the spinal cord and culminates in and around the pituitary gland and the pineal gland in the brain. It is this sushumna nerve, which hosts the kundalini power and facilitates its movement from mooldhara to the sahastrdhara chakra. The onward journey of kundalini beyond sahastrdhara is without the sushumna nerve.

The process of activation of mooldhara has been duly mentioned in chapter 2 of this book. In this section, the concepts of the mantras shall be illustrated, which would aid in activation of this chakra. Post activation of mooldhara chakra, fear, apprehensions or speculations about things, diminishes. The prospects of earnings increase manifold and the business model remains stable. The beej mantras associated with Lord Ganesha are of significant help in activating the mooldhara chakra. This is so, because all the beej mantras for Lord Ganesha are recited in a manner that the breath is held in the throat area while reciting and there is no inhaling or exhaling happening during the recitation.

For awakening of the kundalini, the nature and texture of your thoughts is vital. Your thoughts, even if they are self-centred, should not resonate with reactivity of harming someone or something, may it be humans, flora or fauna. You reserve the right to protect yourself and the perseverance of your success, but not by directly or intentionally harming someone. In spite of this, even if you act consequentially, sanity should prevail within, to trigger the realization of not repeating it in addition to providing solace and comfort to the thing/person who was affected by your action. Additionally, food habits would also witness a distinguishable change with the focus shifting from taste and delicacies to a more balanced and sustainable diet. However, this change should not be viewed as being bereft of the sense of enjoying food, rather, it should be perceived as a preferential shift.

These things do aid in activating the mooldhara chakra, or for that matter, any chakra. However, for the kundalini power to be in attendance in that chakra and exhibit its movement and energy, can only be achieved by focussing on the naad. All these mudras and physical postures create the possibility of stimulations and sensations in the chakras. Nevertheless, for the kundalini to be there, would absolutely depend upon the power of your focus and the ability to relate with the naad. Naad in reality is the sound of kundalini during its movement. Naad is present even when kundalini is in a dormant state. The kind of yog which emphasises on naad, should only be attempted under the supervision of an expert who is well versed with the subject and conscious of the naad so created. In addition, the expert should also be observant and acquainted about the location, significance and energy levels generated by the naad in that chakra. Moreover, if a touch of the healing angle has to be extended, he should be aware of the definitive approach to do so.

Naad is of three major types while progressing in the first six chakras viz. mooldhara, swadishthana, manipura, vishudhi and agya chakra. The naad produced in each of these chakras, apart from having a variation in frequency and amplitude, also varies in pitch pertaining to the energy generated following its movement or travel. The sounds, classified as per the pitch, are as follows:

1. Pashyanti/Pra पशयन्ति/परा
2. Madhyma मध्यमा
3. Vekhri वेखरी

Pashyanti/Pra पशयन्ति/परा: This naad is realized while executing focus-based yog in mooldhara chakra. This naad can be understood as one which the kundalini generates while being in almost a dormant state.

Madhyma मध्यमा: This Naad is experienced when the energy is moving from the swadisthana chakra to the manipura chakra and further towards the anahata chakra. The naad changes when kundalini is awakened and travelling through these chakras, in comparison to what the naad would be when these chakras are activated.

Vekhri वेखरी: This naad germinates when the energy is moving from the anahata chakra to the vishudhi chakra and subsequently to the taalu chakra. The variations in this naad are dependent on the alignment of the lower three chakras.

The physical postures which one should embrace in order to focus on energies at the accurate point are the following:

a. Badhpadam बधपदम
b. Sidh Aasan सिधआसन
c. Vajr Aasan वज्रआसन
d. Swastik Aasan स्वस्तिकआसन

The Principles for Kundalini Awakening

A person can adopt any of these aasan's to perform focus-based yog for a better comprehension and purview of where kundalini is hosted and what is the texture of movement.

The second equally essential thing is the place chosen to perform focus-based yog. Seemingly, the place designated for performing the activity has its own aura, whether you are able to recognise it or not, the effects of the prevailing energies in the sub-stratosphere have a direct impact on your focus-based yog. The place of your choice should decidedly be rich in flora and fauna. Carrying out focus-based yog in a brick and mortar structure may not be fruitful enough to reap the desired results. This is quite critical during the early stages of kundalini awakening or when kundalini hasn't reached the culminating point of the sushumna nerve.

Initially, one may face difficulties in locating the mooldhara chakra. Primarily, this may be due to imbalances in the chakras because of which, the sensations are felt at a point not designated for the mooldhara. Due to this imbalance, the energy shifts its location and is wrongly placed. Consequently, activation of the wrong energy would result in obtaining inaccurate results. Hence, one needs to be more vigilant and observant about the location of the chakras. As illustrated in previous chapters, one has to focus on specified areas only. Even if one experiences the sensations elsewhere, try bringing the sensations to the prescribed location only. Certainly, it cannot be achieved instantly. In very rare cases, the stimulation and the consequent activation can happen much earlier than anticipated.

One should start by focusing on the spine and feel the movement of energy in that area. Just feel the movement without developing any hallucinations or getting carried away by the cognitive memory of the sequel of things. While you may have encountered contrasting notions, based on the experience of others, just be sincere in your focus and observe the developments in the spinal cord area. Post establishing the focus on movement of energy in the spine area, from here onwards, the energy on its own would try moving to glabella and would remain stationed there till a significant improvement is witnessed in the lower four chakras, for this energy to proceed with its journey to the other two chakras, namely, the agya chakra and the sahastrdhara. However, this placement and movement of the energy should not be confused with kundalini. As is the case with kundalini, when it moves, it progresses through all the 114 chakras at one go without any stoppage or halt in between.

In Srimad Bhagavad Gita, there are volumes on kundalini outlining the conversation between Lord Krishna and Arjun. Explicitly, these compositions illustrate the behaviour, relevance, significance and the outcomes of kundalini activation. There are hints in the verses as to what it does, post crossing the sushumna nerve. The interpretation of these verses enshrined in Srimad Bhagavad Gita for the activation of kundalini, are as follows.

One should sit in a padma aasan पद्माआसन with feet facing upwards whilst resting on the joints of leg and the pelvis area. Now, try pressing these joints by applying the force of your feet and keep applying the force in a continual manner. Further, lift your upper torso while maintaining the posture of the padma aasan पद्माआसन. This aasana is also connoted as moolbandh मूलबंध, more popularly known as the vajr aasan वज्रआसन. In this posture, the stress and concentration of the weight would be on lower torso, to be pressed further downwards. At this moment, apaan vayu अपानवायू would tend to return from the back side of the body and commences its flow on the frontal part of the body.

Moving further from this position, with your hands, form droanaakar द्रोणआकार while keeping the spine erect. Now, when you are able to maintain your focus on the spine, an urge to sleep would develop. However, you need to retain the focus to comprehend with the flow of energy in greater volumes, to what you had been experiencing. The energy takes an upward path and starts stimulating the upper chakras, with some protruding outwards and some of them sucking inwards. For example, the manipura chakra will suck in while the swadisthana chakra will protrude out. The anahata chakra will fluctuate in its movement with alternate bouts of squeezing in and protruding out.

Kundalini power by virtue of the bandh and focus-based yog, rises suddenly. However, this rise may not be permanent in nature, as it can slip back to the mooldhara and regain a dormant state and reach manipura chakra. When this transpires, there would be craving for hunger and thirst. Interestingly, this hunger cannot be satisfied by resorting to consumption of anything. Rather, there are specific food articles which would satiate the same. People who are regular and consistent with their focus-based yog, can overcome this urge through the release of extra energy in the body, enabling them to stay longer for focus-based yog.

Whilst reciting the mantras of Lord Ganesha, to stimulate and activate your mooldhara, focus on the bud near the tail bone. Kundalini, resides at this specific point in a dormant state. The beej mantras which are undefined अस्पष्ट, are phonemes (not having any literal meaning), quite capable of stimulating the kundalini.

As explained above, since kundalini moves upwards, the flow of energy is immense and intense, due to which, all the elements through which kundalini passes, get absolved in it. In other words, post the activation of kundalini, behaviourial aspects of the elements are not solitary. Curiously, they merge and blend with each other, resulting in a combination of effects throughout the body. Like, for example, post the activation of swadishtana chakra, element water is quite dominant and if there is an intuition, one would experience tingling sensations in this chakra. Post the awakening of kundalini, this sensation would not only be present in this chakra, but would rather be evenly spread and the flow of water would prohibit the flow of emotions. Nonetheless, it would be aimed at compassion and not passion. Changes in the spine area would also be evident in relation to the behaviour and texture of the hollow bones (these have been explained earlier; and are correlated/recognized as 33 types of GODs in Hinduism). The pre-kundalini awakening behaviour changes all together into different forms, which in yog vashisht is referred to as "leh" लह्. In English language, it can be translated and understood as "dissolving". The things which contribute to dissolving have been connoted as:

1. Rudr रुद्र
2. Laakini लाकिनी
3. Daakini डाकिनी

When kundalini exhibits its influence and there is a sequential transformation in the spine area and the spinal cord, one endures a lot of discomfort. The discomfort can be manifest in the form of high blood pressure, irritability, low blood count, weakness in legs, and inability to cherish companionship. At this stage, a person aspires to remain engaged in focus-based yog and truly cherishes it. Simultaneously, the physical, biological and medical distortions recede, as the body gears up and regains strength to host the awakened kundalini. However, the duration of the aforementioned issues, varies among individuals. Regardless, having these complications is not a certification of having an awakened kundalini. Health related issues may crop up if a person is not doing focus-based yog, specifically targeted towards the awakening of kundalini.

Awakening of kundalini will transform you totally. A pronounced change, encompassing a different format would be visible and one has to be psychologically prepared to undergo this transformation. A lot of things, considered normal prior to awakening of kundalini, would not be much appreciated, post its awakening. However, do not conceive the existing life and societal ethos, to be the ultimate one. Do remember, you are an individual, born alone and will die alone. It is just by choice that you have steered yourself to be part of the conglomerate. Do not dilute your identity just because the others chose not to rise. You have the provision and the possibility to explore and attain it.

The acceptable state of consciousness and transcendental consciousness, are two ends of your consciousness, between whom you are swinging endlessly. Now is the time to make a choice to allow the dominating one. Your perceptions, convictions, emotions and feelings are nothing more than a mere comprehension of things. Just get over them to realise yourself and the immense possibilities that remain undiscovered. This is not an adventure trip but the way life should be. Now is the time to realise and recognise the exploding energies and their corresponding signals that are emerging. By virtue of its profoundness, due respect needs to be extended, ensuring its stability.

The entire process of kundalini awakening comprises of several steps and stages of varying energies, defining as to how kundalini would be traversing through various chakras and hollow bones in the spine. The flow of energy in kundalini, and the flow of energy in ida and pingla ईड़ा और पिंगला, creates ripples in the body of energy which may be felt in the physical body too. If one is observant and fortunate, this flow is continuous in ida and pingla. Nerve sushumna should be assumed as active and augurs well for a "spiritual event" to occur. In the natural course, the breathing patterns would change every hour and the temperature variation of the breath would alter every fourth day.

This change is attributed to the movement of moon, which alters the element of water in the body. The nature of this event will entirely depend on your thought process prevailing. If it is "fabricated and society dependent" and if you have managed to master the silence of brain, the event will ensure further rise in the energies. Else, it will spark off into predictions from your end, likely to turn out true. This may further engulf you in getting stuck in the societal and false "image" building of "being", than really "being" to be "bee-ing" of the energies. It is probable, since you may acquire the powers of clairvoyance, telepathy, and psycho telekinesis (the power to heal someone just by blessings). There is a likelihood that you enter in a phase when you would not like to eat for days together, or you may not demonstrate the appetite for several days and yet won't feel listless even after being deprived of food. Additionally, there are probable chances of slipping into depression or having a personality disorder for a few days.

Some individuals abandon practice and terminate their journey of the spiritual world, following the discomfort experienced in the form of headaches, with a reprieve experienced only while meditating. Also, a few others undergo sleeping disorders resulting in insomnia, prompting them to discontinue the journey.

When kundalini awakens in a yogi, and the consciousness remains constant and consistent, the impulse for sleep and food is non-existent, coupled with no weakness and passion. As observed, having headaches or insomnia is noticeably greater in people having an unsteady sexual life. The reason attributed for this observation pertains to the positioning and activation levels of the swadisthana chakra, than the act of sex per se. One encounters different experiences the time nerves, chakras and ultimately, kundalini gets awakened. Since it is an amalgamation and progression of different energies, one should not scrutinize and miscalculate them to be one. Of course, they do germinate from one source but because of their varying texture and nature, the behaviour is different in and within the body.

In reality, when the awakening materializes, there is a huge upsurge of energy. In the realms of knowledge, there would be experience-based symptoms, but you would fail to explain them to others. The most prudent of the initial experience would be swaying of the body, either to and fro or sideways. You would experience the release of energy in the form of shocks, travelling upwards, normally discharged by the burning sensations in the mooldhara chakra. Other distinct changes likely to be experienced would include, listening to music, hearing others, and seeing unknown faces. At times, you would feel a lightweight body and may visualise a "divine" light. However, I would suggest, that you do not try holding on to these experiences and stay with them. They are just a phase in the journey towards kundalini awakening. These experiences are primal and it is not necessary that everyone would encounter them. If your chakras are already activated, you won't hear or notice them. Do not rank your progress by these kinds of experiences, instead just enjoy the journey.

Going by my personal experience, I can comfortably assert, when the chakras are getting activated. The experiences are not so intense and the changes within the body won't have an impact on your behaviour or physical health being (there may be some temporary alterations). The experiences are generally quite fascinating and pleasing. There would be positive changes in your skin texture, food consumption habits, patience level, and visualization of light and related aspects. However, when sushumna nerve gears to host kundalini within, electric shocks eventualize. These may take the shape of feelings, swaying, blood pressure related issues, seeing or hearing people even when you are alone, insomnia etc. Characteristically, these experiences do not trickle down at a slow pace rather they just come up as an explosion. My reasoning for highlighting this point here is to enlighten people to be firm in their approach while attempting the awakening of kundalini. This endeavour should not be judged as just another task; for it is capable of changing your life forever. Precision and clarity in your roadmap is vital before venturing out on this path. Predominantly, do ensure that the person who is guiding you, has already grasped the treaded path and is a realised master.

Index

A

Aadh Mukhas Aasan, 42
Aakash Chakra, 6
Aarogya Chakra, 6
Aatman, 35
Adhara Lotus, 97
Adho Mukha Aasan, 86
Adho Mukhvkr Aasan, 109
Agni, 25
Agnisthamb Aasan, 85
Agya Chakra, 119, 138, 162
Air, 21
Alaokik Agni, 26
Anahata Chakra, 97, 104, 161
Anand Baal Aasan, 83
Anand Chakra, 6
Anitya Prithvi, 29
Anjaney Aasan, 86
Anxiety Quotient, 15
Apaan Vaayu, 77, 104, 166
Apanaasan, 40, 149
Archetypal Energies, 16
Ardh Chandra Aasan, 64, 127
Ardh Hal Aasan, 40
Ardh Hanuma Aasan, 43
Arjun, 166
Astrological Natal Chart, 4
Avalambaka Kapha, 23
Ayurveda, 29

B

Badhakon Aasan, 84
Bandha, 44
Baudhik Sharir, 37
Beej Mantras, 78, 99, 138
Bhautik Sharir, 37
Bhavnatmak Sharir, 37
Bhrajaka Agni, 26
Bhu Chakra, 6
Bhujang Aasan, 42, 109, 149
Bindu Chakra, 120
Bodhaka Kapha, 23
Brahm Chakra, 5
Breathing, 38, 61, 81, 105, 124, 143
—exercises, 16

C

Chakra Swas Aasan, 106, 129
Chakras (confluence points), 1, 10, 14, 34, 76
—activation, 18
—balancing, 14, 16
—correct analysis, 15
—role, 18
—unblocking, 14
Citrini, 54
Coeliac Plexus, 53
Consciousness, 1

Cosmos, 13
Covid-19, 77
Crown Chakra, 13, 16

D
Dakshin Maargiy, 22, 57
*Devi (shakti/*power*) Puran*, 4
Devtas, 7
Dhyanyog, 18
Digestive Fire, 27
Dominating Chakra, 13
Droanaakar, 166

E
Earth, 21
Eight Stages of Yog, 18
Eight Superpowers, 7
Ekpaskot Aasan, 87
Element Air, 30
Element Earth, 22, 28
Element Ether, 32, 119
Element Fire, 23, 25
Element Space, 22
Emotions, 2
Ether, 21

F
Fingers of the Hand, 20
Fire Element in the Body, 12
Fire, 21
Focus-based Exercises, 16, 44, 66, 111, 130, 150
Focus-based Yog, 165

G
GABA Neuro Transmitters, 11
Gaumukh Aasan, 107, 129
Glabella, 166
Glutamate, 11
God Vahni, 54

H
Hand Formulations, 44, 66, 110, 130, 150
Heart Chakra, 12
Hippocampus Area of the Brain, 11
Hriday Chakra, 5
Hrit Chakra, 101

I
Ida, 8, 9, 139, 141, 162
Indra, 35
Ionic Energy, 16

J
Jallandhar Bandh Yog, 125
Jathraparivart Aasan, 84

K
Kanth Chakra, 6
Kapalbhatti, 62, 144
Kapha, 23
Kapha Dosha, 24
Karma, 6, 100
Kavach Chakra, 6
Kledaka Kapha, 24

Index

Kriyas, 4
Kundalini, 3, 16, 35
  —activation, 3, 10, 18
  —awakening, 159
  —movements, 4
  —power, 2, 3, 5
  —realisation, 18

L
Lom Vilom, 62, 144
Lord Brahma, 37
Lord Ganesha, 36, 162, 167
Lord Krishna, 166
Lord Shiva, 140
Lord Vishnu, 78

M
Maharishi Patanjali, 8
Major Chakras, 11
Manipura Chakra, 53, 57, 58
  —activation, 57
Mantra Recitation, 16, 44, 67, 88, 111, 130, 150
Micro Chakras, 11
Minor Chakras, 11
Mohan Chakra, 6
Moolbandh, 166
Mooldhara Chakra, 34, 80, 162, 165
Mooldhara, 77
Mtsaya Aasan, 108, 126, 146
Mukt Triveni, 161

N
Naabhi Chakra, 5
Naad Kriya, 45, 67, 88, 111, 131
Naad, 163
Nadis, 20
Nath Tradition, 53
Nerves, 9
Nirvaan Chakra, 6
Nitya Prithvi, 29

O
Occult Powers, 120

P
Pachaka Agni, 26
Padma Aasan, 61, 166
Pancha Mahabhutus, 25
Parig Aasan, 107, 128
Parivrata Prasarvkon Aasan, 126
Parmatmam, 35
Parthiv, 28
Personality Traits, 21
Phalaasan, 65, 147
Phemes, 10
Physical Yog, 81, 125, 144
Pineal Gland, 142
Pingala, 8, 9, 139, 141, 162
Pitta, 27
Pitta Dosha, 27
Pituitary Gland, 139
Power of Speech, 5
Praan Vaayu, 103

Pran, 123
Principles of Energy, 1
Prithvi Mudra, 77

R
Rajak Agni, 26
Root Chakra, 3, 12, 76
Rup, 25

S
Sacral Chakra, 12, 76, 78,
Sadhaka Agni, 26
Sahastradhara Chakra, 104, 162
Salbhas Aasan, 42, 66, 148
Samarthya Chakra, 6
Samskaras, 77
Sanshoshan Chakra, 6
Saraswati Rahasyopanishad, 20
Saubhagya Chakra, 6
Self-control, 35
Serpentine Power, 5, 161
Setu Bandh Sarvang Aasan, 41, 125, 146
Seven Chakras, 10
Seven Virtues of the Trunk, 36
Shaap Chakra, 6
Shakti, 1, 2, 4
Shiva, 2
Siddhis, 77, 100
Sidh Aasan, 38, 39, 82
Sidhi Chakra, 6
Sleshaka Kapha, 23

Smaan Vaayu, 104
Solar Plexus Chakra, 60
Solar Plexus, 12
Soul, 18
Sparsh, 31
Spiritual World, 118
Srimad Bhagavad Gita, 166
Stimulation of Root Chakra, 38
Supt Badhakon Aasan, 82
Supt Viraasan, 43
Supta Padangusthasan, 41, 148
Surya Mudra, 88
Sushumna Nadi, 19
Sushumna, 139, 141, 162
Swadishthana Chakra, 5, 75, 161, 167
Swar, 10

T
Taalu Chakra, 6
Tanmatra, 25
Tantra, 22
Tantra Sadhna, 46, 89, 112, 131
Third Eye Chakra, 13
Throat Chakra, 13
Traipura, 138
Trikon Aasan, 64, 126, 147
Types of Nerves, 8

U
Udaan Vayu, 104
Uddiyan Bandh, 62

Ultradian Rhythm, 20
Upavistha Konaasan, 85
Urdv Dhanur Aasan, 110
Ustr Aasan, 108, 148
Utihaprasarvkon Aasan, 65
Uttaasan, 42
Uttan Aasan, 86
Uttanpristh Aasan, 87

V

Vaam Margiy, 22
Vaayu, 30
Varying Sounds, 12, 13
Vashishth Aasan, 65, 147
Vedas, 1, 9, 34, 76, 99
Vedic System, 21
Viprit Virbhadar Aasan, 63, 127, 145
Virbhadhra Aasan, 63, 145
Vishudhi Chakra, 119
Vrittis, 77
Vyaan Vaayu, 103

W

Water Element in the Body, 12
Water Element, 22, 75
Watery Tissues of the Body, 24

Y, Z

Yantra Sadhna, 67, 89, 112, 131
Yog Mudra, 106, 128

Yog Vashsihta, 2
Yukt Triveni, 161